AF879631

The New Vegetarians

Promoting Health and Protecting Life

The New Vegetarians

Promoting Health and Protecting Life

Paul R. Amato, Ph.D.
and
Sonia A. Partridge

Springer Science+Business Media, LLC

Library of Congress Cataloging in Publication Data

Amato, Paul R.
The new vegetarians: promoting health and protecting life / Paul R. Amato and Sonia A. Partridge.
p. cm.
Bibliography: p.
Includes index.

1. Vegetarianism. 2. Vegetarianism—Social aspects. I. Partridge, Sonia A. II. Title.
TX392.A535 1989 88-33636
613.2'62—dc19 CIP

ISBN 978-0-306-43121-0 ISBN 978-1-4899-6004-7 (eBook)
DOI 10.1007/978-1-4899-6004-7

© 1989 Paul R. Amato and Sonia A. Partridge
Originally published by Plenum Press in 1989.
Softcover reprint of the hardcover 1st edition 1989

All rights reserved

No part of this book may be reproduced, stored in a retrieval system, or transmitted in any form or by any means, electronic, mechanical, photocopying, microfilming, recording, or otherwise, without written permission from the Publisher

Preface

We live in a time when meat has never been more abundant. Yet never before have so many people voluntarily passed up a charbroiled steak for a simple plate of beans and rice. Why? Various spokespeople, including doctors, nutritionists, religious teachers, moral philosophers, and animal rights activists, have provided compelling justifications for not eating meat. Although we find these views to be of interest, they are not the primary subject matter of our book. Instead, this book is about ordinary people—the rank and file of the vegetarian movement. We allow vegetarians to speak for themselves and to describe, in their own words, how and why they came to take the first difficult steps in abstaining from animal flesh and the implications this had for their personal and social lives.

We have written this book for several reasons. First, the topic of vegetarianism is a timely and important one. Recent medical research indicates that a high-fat, low-fiber diet centered on meat is a contributing factor in cardiovascular disease—the leading cause of death in the United States today. The typical American diet has also been linked to several forms of cancer, including cancer of the colon, breast, cervix, uterus, ovaries, and prostate. A better understanding of the ways in which vegetarians have reorganized their lives to stop eating meat should make it easier for nonvegetarians to modify their own consumption of animal foods. Second, we find vegetarianism to be an intriguing personal and social phenomenon. Although there are many books available on meatless cooking and vegetarian issues, we know of no other work that shows why people become vegetarians and how this affects their psychological functioning, private lives, and social relationships.

Who would be interested in a book on vegetarians? Those who wish to become vegetarians will find out what to expect, including potential pitfalls as well as benefits. Practicing vegetarians will be able to compare their experiences with those of others. In so doing, they will find that although vegetarians everywhere deal with similar problems, they adopt a variety of solutions and strategies for coping—some of which are more successful than others. Finally, the general reader will find that vegetarians constitute a fascinating subculture, and one that provides insight into topics such as psychological growth, health-promoting behavior, attitude shifts, new lifestyles, and social change.

The material in this book was obtained from three sources. We began by placing notices in vegetarian magazines and newsletters, asking vegetarians to write and tell us about their experiences. Later we mailed questionnaires to vegetarians recruited through a number of organizations. Finally, we conducted personal interviews with vegetarians to gain additional insight into their lives. Some people who are not full-fledged vegetarians, but who had stopped eating certain animal foods such as red meat, were also interviewed. Altogether, we obtained information from over 300 vegetarians, representing a variety of backgrounds, ages, and ethnic groups. Although most of our respondents live in the United States, we also obtained information from vegetarians in Canada, Great Britain, Australia, New Zealand, Europe, and the Middle East. Clearly, vegetarianism is an international movement, and the respondents in our study reflect this. Our procedures generated a rich supply of diverse personal experiences that, taken together, provide a comprehensive picture of the vegetarian lifestyle.

Stereotypes about vegetarians are generally uncomplimentary. It is widely held, for example, that vegetarians are health nuts, members of bizarre religious cults, hippies, or other fringe-dwellers. But our research reveals that most vegetarians today are practical and sensible members of the social mainstream; increasing numbers, in fact, are academics, business people, doctors, lawyers, and other professionals, as well as skilled tradespeople. Vegetarians are also seen as ascetic, skinny, weak, and anemic. However, we show that most vegetarians experience better than average health and typically live physically active, and demanding, lives. Finally, vegetarians are often seen as superficial trend-followers, ready to jump on the latest bandwagon. In contrast, we find that deeply held convictions underlie the diets of most vegetarians.

Vegetarians also differ in their dietary practices. At this point it is a good idea to define some basic terms that distinguish between different types of vegetarians. *Lacto-ovo vegetarians* abstain from flesh of any kind, including beef, veal, pork, lamb, mutton, chicken, and fish. However, they continue to eat eggs and dairy products. Some vegetarians also abstain from eggs but continue to eat dairy products (*lacto-vegetarians*) whereas others abstain from dairy products but continue to eat eggs—particularly free range eggs (*ovo-vegetarians*). *Vegans* do not eat flesh, eggs, or dairy products. In addition, ethical vegans reject the use of many other animal products, such as leather, furs, and soap made from animal fat. People on vegetarian *macrobiotic* diets live mainly on whole grains, sea and land vegetables, beans, and miso. Although some macrobiotic diets allow a small amount of fish (and therefore are not strictly vegetarian), dairy products and eggs are avoided. *Natural hygienists* eat plant foods and reject the use of processed and refined food products. In addition, they believe that certain foods should be combined in particular ways at mealtime; fasting is also part of their regimen. *Raw foodists* eat mainly uncooked foods because they believe that heat destroys many of the enzymes and nutrients. *Fruitarians* eat "fruits" only, although the term is defined broadly to include nuts, seeds, and other foods commonly thought of as vegetables, such as tomatoes and peppers. Finally, some people eat no red meat but continue to eat fish, and perhaps chicken, occasionally. We refer to these people as *semivegetarians*.

Although these categories seem straightforward, they are fuzzy in everyday life. For example, some people call themselves vegetarians, yet continue to eat flesh from fish. Some vegetarians eat animal flesh on rare occasions, such as when visiting family. And some vegans occasionally consume dairy products or eggs (often in baked goods). In this book, we do not adopt a purist view. Instead, we allow people to define for themselves the type of vegetarian they are. We prefer not to banish people from the ranks of vegetarianism for occasional lapses or "heretical" dietary practices. To do so is to confuse logically consistent categories with the actual behavior of people in their everyday lives.

We begin by establishing the context of contemporary vegetarian belief and practice. Vegetarians today draw on a variety of traditions, some of which are thousands of years old. Accordingly, we delineate the various influences that have made contemporary vegetarianism a force to be reckoned with. Then we present the results of our research. We describe people's motives for becoming vegetarians, how they go about making the transition, the implications of these changes for physical and psychological well being, aspects of the vegetarian lifestyle, and the ways in which abstaining from meat affects people's personal lives and social relationships. Finally, we include practical recommendations for people who are considering becoming vegetarians or limiting in a significant way their dependence on animal flesh. Practicing vegetarians will also find suggestions for handling some common problems. We conclude with a look at the future of vegetarianism in the West.

Paul R. Amato
Sonia A. Partridge

Lincoln and San Diego

Acknowledgments

This book was made possible by the enthusiastic and generous support of the vegetarian community. First, we would like to thank our respondents for the time and effort they took to write to us, or to be interviewed, about their experiences as vegetarians. We hope this book does justice to their collective efforts. Second, we would like to thank the many groups who helped to inform vegetarians about our project. These include: The American Vegan Society; *The Animals' Agenda* magazine; The Animals' Crusaders; Animal Liberation, Australia; Baltimore Vegetarians; Behavioural and Political Animal Studies, New Zealand; Boston Vegetarians; East Tennessee Vegetarian Society; Gentle World Community; Govinda's Natural Foods Restaurant, San Diego; Grain Country restaurant, San Diego; House of Afrika restaurant, San Diego; Hygienic Community Network News; International Society for Animal Rights; Jyoti-Bihanga restaurant, San Diego; Kung Food Vegetarian Restaurant, San Diego; L'Chaim Vegetarian Cafe, San Diego; Lehigh Valley Vegetarians; North American Vegetarian Society; Ocean Beach People's Food Co-Op, San Diego; Sacramento Vegetarian Society; The Seventh-Day Adventist Church, Clairemont, San Diego; San Diego Animal Advocates; Psychologists for the Ethical Treatment of Animals; Toronto Vegetarian Association; Uchee Pines Institute; The Vegan Society, England; The Vegan Society of Australia; The Vegetarian Society of D.C.; *Vegetarian Times* magazine; The View from Raspberry Corners; and *Wholistic Living News*. News of our research spread quickly throughout vegetarian networks and many respondents took it upon themselves to recruit their vegetarian friends for our study. We discovered that many groups mentioned our research project in their newsletters, even though we did not directly solicit their assistance. Inevitably, we received help that we are not aware of. We extend our gratitude to all of you. Finally, we would like to thank our editor at Plenum Publishing Corporation, Victoria Cherney, for her insightful advice and encouragement in writing this book.

P. R. A.
S. A. P.

Contents

CHAPTER 1 The Origins of Modern Vegetarianism 1

A Quick History of Vegetarianism 2
The Health Movement 5
Nutrition 6
Coronary Heart Disease 10
Cancer 12
Other Health Issues 14
Religious Movements 15
Hinduism 15
Buddhism 16
Judaism 17
Christianity 17
The Environmental Movement 18
The Animal Liberation Movement 21
The Treatment of Farm Animals 22
Ethical Arguments for Vegetarianism 23
How Different Are Humans and Other Animals? 24
Implications 27
The Movements for Social Justice and Peace 27
Summary 29

CHAPTER 2 Why Do People Become Vegetarians? 31

Locating Vegetarians 31
Characteristics of Vegetarians 32

Reasons for Becoming a Vegetarian *34*
Animal Ethics *35*
Health *38*
Religion *40*
Aesthetics *44*
Personal Growth *45*
World Hunger *47*
Nonviolence *48*
The Environment *49*
A Natural Way of Life *50*
Economics *51*
Social Conformity *52*
Other Motives *52*
Overview of Motives *53*
Changes in Motives over Time *54*
Views of Other Vegetarians *56*
Summary *61*

CHAPTER 3 The Transition to Vegetarianism *63*

Initial Influences *63*
People *64*
Books and Other Literature *68*
Specific Experiences *70*
Organizations *78*
Films *79*
Making the Change *81*
The Quick Change *81*
The Gradual Change *82*
The Benefits of Being Prepared *84*
Just One More Steak *88*
Initial Cravings *88*
Giving In *91*
Feelings about Eating Meat Now *92*
Changes in Vegetarians' Diets *94*
The Change to Veganism *98*

CHAPTER 4 Implications of Vegetarianism for Personal Well-Being 103

Changes in Physical Health 103
Positive Changes 104
Health Problems 113
No Change 115
How Reliable Are People's Reports? 115
Psychological Changes 116
Positive Changes 117
Negative Changes 123
Spiritual Changes 126
Sexual Changes 129
Evaluation of Former Self 131
Summary 135

CHAPTER 5 The Vegetarian Lifestyle 137

So What Do You Eat If You Don't Eat Meat? 137
Alternatives to Flesh 139
Traps for the Unwary 141
Shopping 144
Organic Food or Commercial? 146
Encounters with Meat 147
Fasting 148
Alcohol, Tobacco, and Other Drugs 149
But You Wear Leather, Don't You? 150
Restaurants 153
Traveling 157
Companion Animals 161
Organizational Involvement 163
Vegetarian Communities 165
Dealing with Institutions 166
Employment 168
Summary 173

CHAPTER 6 Relations with Family, Friends, and Acquaintances *175*

Dealing with Family *175*
  Initial Reactions *176*
  Changes over Time *180*
Dealing with Friends and Acquaintances *182*
  Reactions of Friends and Acquaintances *185*
  Vegetarian Friends *185*
  Problems in Socializing *187*
  Dining with Nonvegetarians *190*
  Why Some Meat-Eaters Are So Obnoxious *194*
  Living Arrangements *196*
  The Extended Visit *197*
Stereotypes of Vegetarians *199*
The Missionary Vegetarian *201*

CHAPTER 7 Vegetarianism and Intimate Relationships *205*

Vegetarian Dating Dilemmas *205*
  Vegetarians Only? *207*
  Making Compromises *208*
  Problems in Dating Meat-Eaters *209*
Living Together: Spouses and De Facto Partners *211*
  Vegetarian Couples *211*
  Mixed Couples *213*
  When Relationships Fail *216*
Men, Women, and Vegetarianism *219*
  The Socialization of Men and Women *219*
  Husbands, Wives, and Vegetarianism *220*
Raising Vegetarian Children *222*
  Children's Health *222*
  Children's Diets *225*
  Explaining Vegetarianism to Children *227*
  Parental Strictness *229*
  Problems for Vegetarian Children *232*
  Avoiding Problems *235*
  Long-Term Prospects for Vegetarian Children *237*

CHAPTER 8 Conclusions and Recommendations *239*

Getting Started *241*
Making the Decision *241*
Making the Change *242*
Minimizing Social Conflict *246*
Changing People's Attitudes *250*
Lapsed Vegetarians: Lessons to Be Learned *252*
Lack of Social Support *252*
Inadequate Preparation *255*
Giving in to Cravings *257*
A Weak Commitment *259*
The Future of Vegetarianism *259*

Vegetarian Resources *267*

Organizations *267*
Magazines *268*
Books *268*
Cookbooks *268*
Nutrition *269*

References *271*

Index *277*

The New Vegetarians

Chapter 1

The Origins of Modern Vegetarianism

Vegetarians may be many things, but they are not lonely. A Gallup poll conducted in 1985 for *American Health* magazine found that nearly nine million Americans call themselves vegetarians.[1] In addition, another 40 million adults are eating less meat and more plant foods than in the past. Similarly, a recent consumer study carried out by the National Restaurant Association found that customers are ordering fewer meat dishes and more salads, fresh fruits, and fruit juices than they used to.[2] The number of vegetarian restaurants is also increasing. The "Essential Guide" to vegetarian restaurants published by *Vegetarian Times* magazine in 1987 lists over 1000 entries; a 1978 edition listed only 350.[3] Clearly, the American diet is changing.

The growing mainstream status of vegetarianism is reflected in recent articles in popular magazines. For example, *Newsweek*, in 1986, referred to our healthier eating habits as "vegetarian chic,"[4] and *Time*, in 1988, praised the new vegetarian preferences of health-conscious young adults.[5] Indeed, many individuals have stopped eating meat for health reasons, although some have also been influenced by the animal liberation movement, religious beliefs, concerns about world hunger, or an awareness of the environmental damage caused by livestock production. But whatever their motives, one thing is clear: Vegetarianism can no longer be viewed as a fringe phenomenon.

The Gallup poll also revealed that nearly three fourths of

Americans reject the notion that vegetarianism is merely a passing fad. A look at the historical record reveals that these people are correct. In fact, vegetarianism has a long, although not always illustrious, history in the West. A quick review of this history helps put present-day vegetarianism in perspective.

A QUICK HISTORY OF VEGETARIANISM

It may surprise many people to hear that our early ancestors lived on a semivegetarian diet for several million years. Some anthropologists have fostered the stereotype of "man the hunter," but studies of contemporary "hunter–gatherers" suggest that early humans lived primarily on a diet of plant foods, with supplementation from animal flesh. Studies of tribal Australian aborigines and the Kung-San of South Africa—groups that live under conditions similar to those of our ancestors—show that only about one fourth of their caloric intake derives from animal products. Nuts, seeds, fruits, and vegetables are the staple foods of these groups.[6] A view of early humans as *gatherers* rather than hunters is a more accurate portrayal.

Like most good ideas in the West, vegetarianism was developed by the ancient Greeks.[7] Pythagoras and Porphyry were the best-known practicing vegetarians, but the list of those who advocated a vegetarian diet includes Diogenes, Plato, Epicurus, and Plutarch. The Greeks favored vegetarianism for a variety of reasons. Pythagoras and his followers believed that animals as well as humans have souls, and that after death, an animal may be reincarnated as a human and vice versa. According to this view, animals should not be killed and eaten because all souls have equal worth. Plato, in *The Republic,* described a vegetarian diet as being best suited for his ideal society. Plant foods were preferred, according to Plato, because they promote health and because they require less land to produce than do animal foods. Other Greek thinkers felt that eating animal flesh was naturally repugnant and should be rejected on aesthetic grounds.

The Romans borrowed many ideas from the Greeks, including vegetarianism, and in spite of their penchant for feeding undesirables to the lions, vegetarian ideas survived throughout Roman times. The poet Ovid and the philosopher Seneca are examples of Romans who expounded the cause of vegetarianism.

The fall of Rome and the spread of Christianity across Europe led to a "dark ages" in vegetarian thought. During this time, Christian thinkers such as Saint Augustine and Saint Thomas Aquinas provided intellectual rationalizations for the killing, eating, and general exploitation of animals by humans. They argued that only people have free will, rationality, and souls, and that animals were placed on earth for the convenience and use of humans—views that are still accepted by the majority of Christians today. However, the tradition of vegetarianism was kept alive in dark and dingy Christian abbeys where monks abstained from meat to suppress their animal passions. (The belief that meat consumption is associated with base urges that hinder one's spiritual progress lingers on in the minds of some contemporary vegetarians, as we will see later.) The Benedictines, Trappists, and Cistercians are all examples of monastic orders that practiced vegetarianism for a period of time.

During the 15th century, Europe discovered classical philosophy, art, and science. But it took the Europeans a little longer to rediscover vegetarianism. Leonardo da Vinci, visionary that he was, stood ahead of his time in being a confirmed vegetarian. As he wrote in his notebook:

> I have from an early age adjured the use of meat, and the time will come when men such as I will look upon the murder of animals as they now look upon the murder of men.[8]

The vegetarian "Renaissance" can be said to have occurred during the late 18th and 19th centuries. During this period, Darwin's theory of evolution destroyed the notion that animals are fundamentally different from humans, and in so doing, challenged the religious and philosophical justification for eating them. The new view was that of a continuum of life, with humans and other animals separated in degree, but not in kind.

The implications of the theory of evolution so upset Darwin that he stopped believing in God. He did not, however, give up eating meat.

The new view of animals as distantly related kin was incorporated into the general humanitarian reform movements that occurred at this time. Indeed, many prominent vegetarians and animal welfare promoters were simultaneously involved in other struggles, such as the child welfare and antislavery movements. It was during this period that the first written works on vegetarianism by Europeans appeared. Leo Tolstoy and Percy Bysshe Shelley are examples of 19th-century writers who advocated a meatless lifestyle. For a while, people who abstained from eating flesh were said to be following the "Pythagorean diet." Later, the term "vegetarian" was coined from the Latin word "vegetus," meaning active or vigorous. (The term has misled many into thinking that vegetarians survive only on vegetables—an inaccurate view of vegetarian cuisine.)

Many Christian groups were at the forefront of the burgeoning vegetarian movement. The Bible Christian Church, founded by William Cowherd in 1809 in Manchester, England, played a major role in advocating and furthering the cause of vegetarianism. Members believed that Christ's teachings of mercy should be extended to animals as well as to people. They also believed that a vegetarian diet was healthier than one based on meat and that Christians have a duty to maintain good health in order to do God's work. Members of this group later formed the Vegetarian Society in 1847—the first secular vegetarian organization in the West. They disseminated information in the form of essays and lectures and taught that the adoption of vegetarianism would lead to universal brotherhood, an increase in happiness, and a more civilized society. This group still exists and is presently known as the Vegetarian Society of the United Kingdom.

The movement was carried on into the 20th century by vegetarian societies working at the grass-roots level, religious groups such as the Seventh-Day Adventists, and prominent figures such as George Bernard Shaw and Mohandas Gandhi. Vegetarian organizations formed in most Western countries, and newsletters, books, and other publications promoting the diet became common. In 1908 the International Vegetarian Union was formed, with its main function being to organize conferences at which vegetarians from around the world meet and share information. The union continues to be active today.

This orderly but gradual progression might have continued indefinitely had it not been for the social upheavals of the 1960s and 1970s. At this point in time, a variety of influences converged that had major implications for the course of vegetarianism: a new awareness of the importance of diet in maintaining health, an interest in Eastern philosophy and religion, a concern over the degradation of the environment through human "progress," a politically active stance in support of the rights of oppressed groups, the emergence of the peace movement, and a utopian belief in a perfectible society. All of these social trends provided pathways for new converts to the vegetarian cause. Out of this melange, the modern era of vegetarianism emerged.

In the remainder of this chapter, we review these sources of influence in some detail. Because they provide the social context for contemporary vegetarian beliefs and lifestyles, understanding a little about them makes it possible to appreciate better the experiences of individual vegetarians described later.

THE HEALTH MOVEMENT

The belief that a vegetarian diet is healthier than a diet based on flesh is not a recent idea. Certain Greek thinkers advocated vegetarianism for health reasons, as we noted. And religious groups formed in Victorian times, such as the Seventh-Day Adventists, believed that meat is harmful to the body, and hence, to the soul. Nevertheless, the notion of a link between meat consumption and health was given a boost during the 1960s, which saw an increased demand for "natural" foods and an interest in preventative means of maintaining health through diet and exercise.

At the same time that alternative health practitioners were stressing the importance of a diet based on whole, unprocessed plant foods, the results of studies conducted by academic researchers were beginning to shake up established medical thinking. Traditional opinion had always held that vegetarianism is a risky business. But the data, as they began to accumulate, were surprising: not only were all the essential nutrients present in a meatless diet, but well-fed vegetarians, as a group, had fewer health problems and lived longer than did meat-eaters.

Nutrition

Dietetic studies show that the great majority of vegetarians have nutritionally sound diets.[9] The results of these studies led the United States National Academy of Sciences–National Research Council (the same group that publishes the RDA figures for vitamins and minerals) to declare in 1974 that a well-planned vegetarian diet is safe.[10] (Exceptions were made, of course, for extremely restricted diets, such as one based entirely on brown rice and tea.) Similarly, in a 1988 position paper, the American Dietetic Association states, "Vegetarian diets are healthful and nutritionally adequate when appropriately planned."[11] Of course, the American Dietetic Association points out that meat-eaters also need to plan their diets with care to ensure optimal health.

But do vegetarians get enough protein? This is probably the most frequently asked question about meatless diets, as any vegetarian will testify. Just how much protein a person should have is an issue of some disagreement among experts. The National Research Council recommends one of the highest levels: 56 grams a day for a 154-pound adult man and 44 grams a day for a 120-pound adult woman.[12] As it turns out, the majority of Americans get too much protein—nearly twice what their bodies can use, based on the National Research Council figures. Excess protein confers little benefit; it is simply excreted from the body. (In fact, a high consumption of protein has been shown to place a strain on the kidneys and lead to calcium loss, as we discuss later.) Although vegetarians eat less protein than do meat-eaters, they readily get as much as they need from nonflesh sources. Even vegans, who eat only plant foods, get more than the maximum recommended level.[13]

Where do vegetarians get their protein? Vegetarians who consume eggs or dairy products get plenty of protein from these sources. For example, a two-egg omelette served with 3½ ounces of cottage cheese and two pieces of whole wheat toast provides 33 grams of protein. But animal products are by no means necessary. Because protein contains about 4 calories per gram, a 154-pound adult male who eats 2500 calories a day needs to consume 9 percent of his calories every day in the form of protein to meet the National Research Council recommendation. Inspection of published food tables reveals that most grain products, legumes, nuts, seeds, and vegetables contain *more* than 9 percent of their calories in the form of protein. For example, in terms of calories, oatmeal is 15 percent protein, lentils are 29 percent protein, peas are 26 percent protein, almonds are 12 percent protein, sunflower seeds are 17 percent protein, potatoes are 11 percent protein, and broccoli is 45 percent protein.[14] And these foods are by no means atypical. Protein, it seems, is everywhere. For example, 7 ounces of tofu served with one cup of cooked brown rice and a small stalk of broccoli provides 25 grams of protein. Assuming that you eat a range of plant foods every day, if you get enough calories, you are almost certain to get enough protein.

derived from animals, contain less of the essential amino acids that make up protein. Based on this idea, it was once thought that two or more plant foods with relatively high quantities of particular amino acids had to be combined within a meal to yield proteins as "complete" as those found in meat. For example, the amino acids in rice and beans were said to complement each other and form a complete protein when served together. Frances Moore Lappé, in her 1971 book, *Diet for a Small Planet,* helped to popularize this notion.

However, although the belief in protein complementarity is widespread, even among vegetarians, its importance appears to have been greatly exaggerated. The American Dietetic Association points out that a plant-based diet provides adequate amounts of all amino acids if a variety of foods are eaten over the course of a day. They state, "It is not necessary that complementation of amino acid profiles be precise and at exactly the same meal, as the recently popularized 'combined proteins theory' suggested."[15] Indeed, the theory of protein complementarity has made a strict vegetarian diet seem unnecessarily difficult and complex. Lappé herself, in the 1981 version of the same book, modified her earlier view and stated that with a reasonably varied diet, the conscientious combining of plant proteins is not required.[16]

Another common misconception is that protein makes people strong and is necessary for doing hard work. In fact, the major function of protein is to create and replace body tissue, such as skin, muscle, and bone. It is complex carbohydrates, such as grains, legumes, and vegetables, that provide energy—not meat. Consistent with this notion, sports records suggest that vegetarian athletes tend to surpass meat-eating athletes in events that require endurance, such as running, swimming, and tennis.[17] Presumably, this is due to the fact that the calories they might otherwise obtain from meat and fat (which are high in calories) are replaced with energy-providing complex carbohydrates.

Lacto-ovo-vegetarians and lacto-vegetarians generally have little trouble obtaining adequate levels of other nutrients. Some nutritionists have warned that vegetarians who exclude *all* animal products from their diets run some risk of deficiencies in iron, riboflavin, zinc, calcium, vitamin D, and vitamin B-12.[18] This may particularly affect pregnant women and children—people whose nutritional needs are relatively great. However, good plant sources exist for iron, riboflavin, zinc, and calcium.[19] Iron can be obtained from peas, beans, tofu, seeds, nuts, and green leafy vegetables. Riboflavin can be obtained from green leafy vegetables, mushrooms, broccoli, and almonds. Zinc can be obtained from nuts, legumes, and whole grains. And calcium can be obtained from green leafy vegetables, cabbage, sesame seeds, almonds, and soybeans. Strict vegetarians should have relatively little trouble obtaining these nutrients if they eat a well-balanced diet (the same principle, of course, holds for meat-eaters).

Vitamin D is one nutrient not present in plant foods. But it is also uncommon in foods of animal origin, except for fish. Most people obtain dietary vitamin D from fortified milk, so vegetarians who consume milk have little difficulty in obtaining adequate quantities. Of course, vitamin D can be readily synthesized in the human body from sunlight. In a temperate climate, about 10 minutes of exposure to the sun per day for people with light skin and 40 minutes for people with dark skin is sufficient.[20] However, black vegans, particularly children, who are exposed to the sun infrequently may run some risk of a deficiency. (This is because their skin pigmentation decreases the absorption of sunlight.) For this reason, they might wish to supplement their diets with vitamin D; certain brands of soy milk are fortified with vitamin D and can be used for this purpose.

Vitamin B-12 is also not available in the plant kingdom, and hence, is of concern to vegans. (B-12 is found in milk and eggs, however, so it is readily available to lacto-ovo-vegetarians.) The vitamin is synthesized by microflora living in the digestive tracts of animals and is readily available in meat and dairy products. Vitamin B-12 is necessary for blood cell formation and nervous system functioning, and deficiencies can lead to several disorders, including megaloblastic anemia and pernicious anemia. In theory, vegans should be prime candidates for these problems. In fact, however, vitamin B-12 deficiencies are relatively uncommon.[21] Richard Bargen, a medical doctor, reviewed all the studies of B-12 deficiencies reported in the medical literature up until the mid 1970s and found virtually no cases of deficiencies in well-fed vegans.[22] (Deficiencies were found, however, in vegans on restricted diets.)

There are several explanations for this apparent paradox. First, people need extremely small amounts of this nutrient, and quantities are stored in the body for years. Small amounts of B-12 have been detected in the soil, in water, and on the surfaces of many plants; these are likely to be ingested occasionally and to contribute toward the B-12 nutriture of people.[23] Second, microflora synthesize a good deal of B-12 in the human colon, but this occurs too low in the intestinal tract to be absorbed. However, these microflora have also been detected in the small intestine (where nutrients can be absorbed), so it is possible that significant amounts are generated within the human body itself.[24] Third, some foods frequently eaten by vegetarians, such as tempeh (fermented soy beans) and nutritional yeast, contain B-12 (although some of this B-12 may not be in a form usable by the body). Of course, vegans who wish to avoid the risk of a deficiency can simply add a cobalamin supplement to their diets.

Before concluding our discussion of nutrition, it is necessary to point out the *benefits* of a vegetarian diet. Meat contains a high proportion of its calories in the form of fat. Yet, most Americans presently get too many of their calories from fat. And although meat is a good source of protein, most Americans, as pointed out above, get more than they need. So many of the calories in meat are, for all practical purposes, wasted. When people replace the calories in their diets from meat with calories obtained from fruits, vegetables, legumes, and grains, they get more nutrients on a calorie-for-calorie basis. Meat also contains a good deal of cholesterol and no fiber; plant foods, in contrast, contain no cholesterol and a good deal of fiber. As one would expect, vegetarians, compared with meat-eaters, consume less saturated fat, less cholesterol, and more fiber—all of which represent significant dietary advantages. In fact, several studies show that lacto-ovo-vegetarians and vegans attain most of the currently recommended dietary goals *better* than do omnivores.[25] When mother said, "Eat your vegetables," she knew what she was talking about.

Coronary Heart Disease

Coronary heart disease is the leading killer in the United States today, resulting in about three quarters of a million deaths per year. Cross-national evidence has long suggested that our dependence on animal foods might be a factor. For example, countries with the highest consumption of animal fats include New Zealand, Australia, Finland, and the United States. These countries also have the world's highest rates of heart disease mortality.[26] In contrast, the Japanese traditionally ate a low-fat diet, and the rate of coronary heart disease there has been only about one tenth of that in the United States. However, Japanese consumption of fat has doubled in recent years, and, correspondingly, the rate of heart disease has increased fourfold.[27]

According to the American Heart Association (AHA), the three major risk factors in heart disease are high blood cholesterol, high blood pressure, and smoking. (Four secondary risk factors are diabetes, lack of exercise, obesity, and a family history of heart disease.) In 1985, the AHA took into account recent medical findings and stated:

> We have good evidence that most people . . . can reduce a major risk of having a heart attack by following a cholesterol lowering plan. . . . Foods of plant origin, such as fruits, vegetables, grains, nuts and seeds, contain no cholesterol. These foods are highly recommended.[28]

Although absent in plant foods, cholesterol is present in meat, poultry, seafood, dairy products, and eggs. Cholesterol is the main component of the plaque that builds up in arteries, causing atherosclerosis. Saturated fats also increase cholesterol levels, so the AHA has recommended cutting back on these as well. Saturated fats are primarily found in animal products, although a few plant foods, such as coconut oil, are also high in content. The AHA has recommended in their dietary guidelines that beans, lentils, tofu, and other plant foods be substituted for meat in main courses at least a few times a week.

What are the implications for vegetarians? Not surprisingly, nutritional studies have shown that vegetarians, compared with meat-eaters, consume less cholesterol and saturated fat, and correspondingly, have lower levels of serum cholesterol and triglycerides (fats).[29] Studies have also found that vegetarians, compared with meat-eaters, have lower rates of atherosclerosis and fatal heart disease.[30] (Some studies have shown, as one would expect, more benefits for vegans than for lacto-ovo-vegetarians.) Although these beneficial effects of a vegetarian diet are linked to the relatively low consumption of cholesterol and saturated fats, studies have also found that vegetarians have lower blood pressure and lower weight than do meat-eaters—two other protective factors in heart disease.

Cancer

As with coronary heart disease, cross-national evidence suggests that our high rate of cancer in the West is linked to diet. For example, India, Mexico, and Africa all have relatively low rates of cancer, and people in these regions consume relatively little meat and a good deal of fiber. In contrast, Argentina, which has a higher rate of beef consumption than the United States, also has higher rates of cancer of the colon and breast. The Japanese traditionally ate little meat and also had low rates of certain cancers, such as colon cancer; however, among those moving to the United States and adopting a meat-centered diet, rates of colon cancer have increased.[31]

A report issued by the U.S. Department of Health and Human Services (USDHHS) estimated that 35 percent of cancer deaths are related to the things we eat.[32] To place this figure in perspective, 30 percent of cancer deaths in the United States every year are due to smoking. The USDHHS report stated, "A diet low in fiber and high in fat, with few fruits and vegetables, or whole grain products, increases the risk of certain cancers."[33] In particular, diet is linked to cancer of the colon–rectum, breast, prostate, and endometrium (the lining of the uterus). Of all cancer killers, cancer of the breast is the second most common among women (after lung cancer), whereas cancer of the colon–rectum is the second most common among men (after lung cancer) and the third most common among women. Because of this, the American Cancer Society has recommended decreasing the proportion of calories in the diet from fat and increasing the amount of dietary fiber from whole grains, legumes, and vegetables.[34]

Although the links between diet and cancer are well established, the precise physiological mechanisms relating the two are not well understood. A high-fat, high-protein, low-fiber diet appears to increase the risk of colon cancer for several reasons. Bacteria in the bowel modify dietary fat into carcinogenic substances that promote the growth of colon tumors. In addition, dietary fiber, as it moves through the colon, helps to dilute the carcinogenic material and reduces its exposure to the bowel walls. The fat in meat also appears to stimulate the production of prolactin in women—a hormone involved in lactation. Some studies have found a link between prolactin levels and cancer of the breast. In addition, vegetarians, compared with meat-eaters, consume larger amounts of fruits and vegetables known to have a protective role against cancer. In particular, carotene (found in carrots, spinach, yams, peaches, and apricots) and vitamin C (found in broccoli, brussels sprouts, cabbage, and oranges) appear to decrease the risk of certain cancers.[35]

Although animal fat is dangerous, it is not the only risk factor in meat. The American Institute for Cancer Research warns that barbecued meat and fish contain mutagens—substances that have been shown to induce cancer by damaging the DNA in human cells.[36] On an outdoor grill, fat from meat drips onto hot coals and forms benzopyrene which is then carried on the smoke and deposited on the meat. Broiling or frying meat can also form carcinogenic substances if the food is charred. Processed foods such as ham, sausage, bologna, frankfurters, and salami are treated with sodium nitrate and sodium nitrite—substances known to be carcinogenic—to retard the growth of bacteria and to make the meat appear fresher than it really is. In addition, most animals raised for slaughter are fed growth stimulants and hormones, many of which are believed to be cancer-inducing.

Given these considerations, we would expect vegetarians, with their diets low in fat, high in fiber, high in fresh fruits and vegetables, and low in charbroiled and processed foods, to have lower rates of cancer than meat-eaters. This is precisely what research shows. Compared with meat-eaters, vegetarians have lower rates of cancer of the colon–rectum, breast, prostate, uterus, and lungs.[37]

Other Health Issues

We have already noted that vegetarians have lower rates of coronary heart disease and some forms of cancer than do meat-eaters. Other studies have found that vegetarians also have relatively few problems with diabetes, osteoporosis, hemorrhoids, arthritis, liver disease, kidney disease, and obesity.[38] The case of osteoporosis—a gradual loss of bone density—is of particular interest. Since the mid-1980s, women have been encouraged to consume more dietary calcium, primarily in the form of milk, to guard against this affliction. Yet, overconsumption of protein appears to be a factor in the disease. Excess protein, it appears, causes calcium to leach from the body. In fact, studies show that a 50 percent reduction in the amount of protein consumed results in a 50 percent reduction in the amount of calcium excreted through the kidneys.[39] Vegetarians appear to be protected from osteoporosis because their moderate, rather than excessive, consumption of protein minimizes calcium loss.

Vegetarians are also less likely than meat-eaters to have an encounter with salmonellosis. The U.S. Food and Drug Administration estimated that in 1985, four million Americans were afflicted with salmonellosis, and of these, 35,000 were hospitalized, 1000 died, and 120,000 were left with chronic crippling diseases such as arthritis.[40] Salmonella bacteria, which are found in the feces of animals, wind up in meat when animals are slaughtered and processed (carcasses are often spattered with intestinal matter when disemboweled). A government study conducted in 1987 revealed that 40 percent of chickens sold to consumers were contaminated with salmonella bacteria. (Eggs can also be contaminated with salmonella bacteria, so lacto-ovo-vegetarians continue to run some risk of the illness.)

Studies clearly show that vegetarians live longer than meat-eaters.[41] In a country as health-conscious as the United States, this sort of information is not going unheeded. As the health advantages of vegetarianism become more widely known in the community, an increasing number of people are responding by restricting their consumption of flesh and increasing their consumption of plant foods. Currently, health benefits serve as one of the best selling points for attracting new converts to vegetarianism.

RELIGIOUS MOVEMENTS

During the 1960s—which was a rather introspective period—many people became intrigued with religion and philosophy, particularly forms originating in the East. Because vegetarianism is a central component in many systems of Eastern thought, this helped to inject a new and somewhat exotic spirit of vegetarianism into the West. Others turned to familiar religions—Christianity and Judaism—and discovered that vegetarian elements had been there all along.[42]

Hinduism

Many people in the West were introduced to Hindu ideas through the music of George Harrison and the Beatles. For young people searching for an alternative way of expressing spiritual feelings, Hinduism offered colorful rituals and an elaborate set of metaphysical beliefs that seemed to fit the times. The basis of vegetarianism in Hinduism is the belief that all living creatures possess souls; when death occurs, the soul is reborn in another form. The law of karma states that the good and the bad that people do during their lifetimes determine whether they will be reborn in a higher or a lower form. For example, a person who behaves unethically may be reborn as a dog or a reptile. On the other hand, a person who behaves ethically may be reborn into a higher status, perhaps as a Brahman. According to this view, to kill animals unnecessarily is wrong because this interrupts their spiritual journeys, forces them to suffer another rebirth, and generally upsets the cosmic scheme of things.

Many people at the time had their first taste of vegetarian food courtesy of the International Society for Krishna Consciousness (ISKCON)—one of the most successful and conspicuous of the Hindu sects operating in the West. ISKCON not only operates a chain of low-cost lacto-vegetarian restaurants, but also puts on regular free feasts for the public at local temples. Interestingly, ISKCON followers believe that plants also have souls, so killing them is problematic as well, although not as serious as killing animals. However, if plant foods are offered up to Krishna before being eaten, bad karma can be avoided.

Buddhism

Buddhism—particularly in the form of Zen—first attained a degree of popularity in the West during the 1950s beatnik era. Later, Zen was absorbed into the counterculture of the 1960s, and a number of Zen monasteries and centers opened for Western adherents. One particular vegetarian diet, known as the macrobiotic diet, derives its inspiration from Japanese Zen Buddhism.

Vegetarianism in Buddhism is based on the doctrine of compassion and noninjury to all living things. As in Hinduism, it is believed that through reincarnation, cattle may become people and vice versa. It is also believed, as in Hinduism, that through a life of good work and meditation, a person can achieve enlightenment and be released from the cycle of death and rebirth. Because all living things may one day come to realize their perfect "Buddha nature," all life is considered to be sacred.

The implications of these teachings for vegetarianism have produced a centuries-old debate among Buddhists. The Buddha himself was a lacto-vegetarian. Yet, many Buddhists believe that it is acceptable to eat meat from an animal that has not been slaughtered specifically for one's own meal (it may have been slaughtered for someone else's meal, however). The Theravada Buddhists, in fact, teach that the Buddha died from eating a piece of contaminated pork. As the story goes, the Buddha was invited to dine with one of his devotees. When the Buddha discovered that he was being served pork, he ate a piece, so as not to offend. This was a mistake, and the Buddha died. Mahayana Buddhists dispute the story and claim the Buddha died after eating a mushroom. They insist that flesh-eating is contrary to the Buddha's teachings. However, this form of Buddhism, which later spread from India to China and Japan (and eventually to the West), has not led to a thoroughgoing vegetarian tradition. Instead, the Buddha's teachings have been honored more in principle than in practice.

Judaism

Judaism contains prohibitions on some animal foods, such as pork and blood. However, the Biblical teaching that God gave people dominion over all living things, and that animals were placed on earth for the use of humans, is hardly fertile ground for the growth of a compassionate vegetarian ethic. Consequently, there has never been a strong tradition of vegetarianism in Judaism. Nevertheless, some Jews have pointed out that a scriptural basis exists for a vegetarian philosophy. For example, the Hebrew bible indicates that flesh was not eaten in the Garden of Eden; it was only after the great flood that it was permitted. (Ironically, it seems that Noah and his family saved the animals on the ark only to eat them later.) Other passages from Genesis suggest that animals possess souls, should be treated kindly, and should be allowed to rest, along with people, on the Sabbath.

A contemporary group, the Jewish Vegetarian Society, currently has branches in many countries and publishes a magazine, *The Jewish Vegetarian*. An editorial by Philip Pick entitled "What is Jewish about Vegetarianism?" argued that Judaism requires an attitude of kindness toward animals. Because of the cruelty involved in factory farming and in the slaughter of animals, animal flesh cannot be considered kosher. Therefore, eating meat can be seen to be against the spirit, if not the word, of Jewish law.

Christianity

As was the case for Judaism, mainstream Christianity never generated a strong vegetarian tradition. Jesus himself appears to have taught that diet is unimportant, and he broke with the elaborate dietary rules of Judaism. Although it is not clear whether Jesus ate flesh, the New Testament tells us that on one occasion he miraculously multiplied fishes and loaves to feed the masses, so we can presume that he at least approved of eating fish. Church officials later consolidated the view that only humans have souls, and in so doing, put the official stamp of approval on the killing and eating of animals. The Protestants, although they disagreed with Catholics over a good many things, generally concurred that all foods, including meat, are acceptable if taken in moderation.

However, there are exceptions. During medieval times, several monastic orders, such as the Trappists, refrained from eating meat, as we saw earlier. There are about 3000 Trappist monks in the world today, and although vegetarianism is no longer mandatory, most continue to adhere to a meatless diet. In fact, Trappists in the United States generate most of their income by producing and selling vegetarian food—particularly baked goods—to the larger community.

The Seventh-Day Adventists are another vegetarian Christian group. In the 19th century, Ellen White (Harmon), the sect's founder, taught that the body is God's temple, and as such, should not be abused through the use of alcohol, tobacco, or meat. She also advocated the use of natural, unrefined foods. Today there are about two million Seventh-Day Adventists in the United States, and although it is not necessary to be a vegetarian to belong, about one half follow a lacto-ovo-vegetarian diet (a small proportion are vegan). Consistent with their emphasis on health, the Seventh-Day Adventists operate numerous clinics, sanitariums, and hospitals, as well as a medical school and research center in Loma Linda, California. They also produce a variety of vegetarian foods for sale, specializing in products that simulate the texture and appearance of meat.

THE ENVIRONMENTAL MOVEMENT

Most people are aware of the deleterious effects of the automobile and heavy industry on the ecology of our planet. But few are aware that meat production has contributed greatly to environmental deterioration.

As Frances Moore Lappé pointed out in *Diet for a Small Planet*, there have been two population explosions in the 20th century: people in Third World countries and livestock in Western countries.[43] This increase in the number of livestock has been accompanied by a trend for livestock to spend all or part of their lives in feedlots where they eat large quantities of grain and soybeans. (Cattle, for example, are fed about 22 pounds every day.) Feeding large numbers of animals in this fashion requires an enormous agricultural output. In fact, one half of the agricultural output of the United States every year goes to feed livestock.[44]

Feedlot agriculture has placed a strain on our natural resources and the quality of our environment. For one thing, water resources are being squandered at an alarming rate. One half of the water consumed in the United States is used in livestock production.[45] (This includes water used directly by livestock and water used for the irrigation of crops to feed livestock.) Presently, about 2500 gallons of water are required to produce one pound of beef. This is an inefficient use of water to produce food, given that it takes about 15 times as much water to produce one pound of protein from beef as it does from soybeans. Not surprisingly, there is evidence that the heavy demand for water by the meat industry is leading to the depletion of unrenewable underground water reserves.

Approximately seven billion tons of topsoil are eroded every year in the United States. With the loss of topsoil, the fertility of the land and its yield are decreased. As it turns out, the majority of soil erosion is linked to overgrazing or the growing of food for livestock.[46] As they graze, cattle clear the land of vegetation and trample the ground, leaving the soil easily eroded by water and wind. Under natural conditions, the densities of ranging animals cause little harm, but the desire for profit has led owners to graze cattle in densities that frequently result in long-term soil damage. Consequently, overgrazing has been the major cause of desertification, both in the United States and around the world. Large numbers of cattle are also grazed on public lands, including national parks, recreational areas, and military reservations—a practice that places our supposedly protected lands at risk.[47] In addition, corn, soybeans, and other crops grown in large quantities to feed livestock are among those that cause the most damage to the soil. Production of these crops could be lessened if they were not required for fattening up animals in feedlots. Furthermore, the clearing of land for livestock agriculture has resulted in massive deforestation. This loss of forest land has contributed further to soil erosion and the depletion of water reserves.

One might wonder what happens to the two billion tons of manure produced annually by farm animals. Much of the nitrogenous wastes turns into soluble ammonia and nitrates which leach through the soil and contaminate the groundwater. This runoff encourages the growth of algae that deplete the water of oxygen and result in the death of aquatic life. Manure, however, is not the only problem. The dumping of unusable waste products such as viscera, grease, and other by-products of the meat industry—much of which winds up in our water—is a cause for concern. The enormous quantity of waste generated gives the animal food industry the distinction of being one of the world's largest polluters of water.[48]

Our wildlife has also suffered as a direct consequence of livestock production, for the clearing of large tracts of land and forests for agriculture has reduced the size and range of natural habitats. This problem is particularly acute in the Amazon basin in Brazil where land is being cleared at a phenomenal rate for the grazing of cattle. (One might assume that the resulting beef would help to feed the hungry people of Brazil, but most of the meat winds up in hamburgers in American fast-food restaurants. Except for a few wealthy landowners, the local people receive little benefit.[49]) Grazing animals alter the ecological balance, placing wild plants and animals at risk. This behavior underestimates our dependence on the ecosystem and reflects an attitude that wildlife and forests stand in the way of progress. An Australian expression aptly summarizes this view: if it moves, shoot it; if it doesn't, cut it down.

The damage inflicted on our environment by large-scale livestock production is, of course, unnecessary. Frances Moore Lappé described livestock as "protein factories in reverse." As she pointed out, 16 pounds of grain and soy fed to a cow yield only one pound of meat in return. And compared with the one pound of meat it produces, the 16 pounds of grain have 21 times more calories, 8 times more protein, and a good deal more fiber.[50] In the United States alone, 124 million tons of soybeans and grain are lost every year through livestock production, averaging out to one cup of grain for every human on earth every day.

Given the inequities of food distribution in the world, it seems unlikely that the United States could literally feed the world with its agricultural output. However, it is clear that the solution to the problem of hunger in the Third World does not include an increase in livestock production. Meat consumption is a luxury available to people in affluent countries—and one that is bought at the price of environmental damage and poor health. The world's population cannot be supported on the high-meat diet common in Western countries; instead, Third World countries will need to adopt the least wasteful method of food production. The world will only be fed when a large proportion of its population lives as vegetarians.

THE ANIMAL LIBERATION MOVEMENT

The 1960s saw the rise of the civil rights and feminist movements. During this time, many young people were unwilling to accept the unequal treatment of minorities and women in favor of white males. This, coupled with a concern about ecology, led some to consider not only our treatment of wildlife, but our treatment of farm and laboratory animals as well. A key development was the publication in 1975 of Peter Singer's book, *Animal Liberation*. This book shocked many people with its account of the mistreatment of animals in modern factory farms and laboratories. Singer also provided philosophical and ethical arguments for extending the right to equal and fair treatment to animals. These arguments were persuasive and helped to lay the foundation for many of the animal rights groups in existence today.

The Treatment of Farm Animals

Over four billion farm animals are slaughtered in the United States every year.[51] (This excludes fish, ducks, and deer.) In the quest for higher profits, most chickens, cattle, and pigs in the United States and England are raised intensively on "factory farms." Living conditions on these factory farms have pushed animal endurance to the limit. Many of these practices would be illegal if pet owners treated their cats or dogs this way.[52]

What are these conditions like? Animals are generally confined in overcrowded and unsanitary warehouses or feedlots. Egg-laying chickens are housed in batteries—large rows of cages stacked four or more high—where as many as four chickens are crammed in a space no larger than one square foot. Many sows and milking cows are kept restrained for most of their lives in isolated cubicles where they are unable to turn around. Veal calves—which are a by-product of the dairy industry—are kept tethered in unlit stalls with no bedding and in which they are unable to lie down properly. They are also fed iron-deficient diets to produce anemia so that their flesh will remain pale.

Farm animals raised intensively are deprived of normal social contact, leading to the development of unnatural pathological behavior. For example, the overcrowding of battery hens upsets dominance hierarchies and results in aggression and cannibalism. To prevent injury, the birds are debeaked—a procedure that requires cutting through sensitive tissue similar to the quick in human fingernails. Pigs are particularly intelligent and sensitive animals; yet sows with litters are kept restrained on concrete floors to prevent them from killing their offspring. Pigs also develop neurotic behaviors, such as grinding their teeth on the metal bars in their stalls.

In addition to their conditions of confinement, other farm practices result in animal suffering. For example, cattle and pigs undergo a series of painful procedures without the benefit of anesthesia, such as branding, dehorning, docking (removing part of the tail), and notching of ears. And the hauling of animals over long distances in open trucks causes many to die of heat exhaustion or of the cold.

The slaughtering process invariably involves pain, although some practices are worse than others. The use of electrical stunning to knock an animal unconscious before having its throat cut is the least painful method of slaughtering, but many animals are not afforded this small courtesy. The killing of chickens, for example, is often done without stunning. Instead, the birds are hung upside down on an assembly line and are passed by a blade that cuts their jugular veins. The chickens are then submersed in vats of scalding water. This method has some drawbacks for odd-sized birds, for many miss the blade and go to the scalding tank alive. Many people believe that kosher methods of slaughter are more humane than nonkosher methods, but this is a misperception. Kosher slaughtering involves hoisting the animal into the air by a back limb (often resulting in dislocation of joints) and cutting the throat while the animal is fully conscious. Animals also suffer in the slaughterhouse before they reach the slaughtering platform. The smell of death stirs fear in animals and necessitates the use of electrical prods and other coercive means to get them to enter the chutes. For many animal rights supporters, the very idea of humane slaughter is a contradiction in terms.

Ethical Arguments for Vegetarianism

In *Animal Liberation* and in subsequent publications, philosopher Peter Singer presented a utilitarian argument for vegetarianism based on the principle of equality of interest. Singer argued that sentient creatures (those with perception and the ability to feel pain) should be afforded equality of interest with humans. In a situation in which there is a conflict of interests, utilitarianism attempts to find solutions that allow the most favorable balance of good (pleasure) and bad (pain). Considering that meat-eating is unnecessary for human health, the pleasures enjoyed by humans are trivial compared with the suffering inflicted on animals. Accordingly, the best balance of good over bad can be achieved through vegetarianism. On this basis, Singer suggested that one should not eat animal flesh, dairy products, or eggs.[53]

Since the publication of Singer's book, a number of other philosophical positions have been advanced. Tom Regan, in *The Case for Animal Rights,* has gone further than Singer in arguing that, regardless of the costs and benefits for animals and humans, animals have certain fundamental rights similar to those we ascribe to humans. According to Regan, animals, as well as humans, can be considered to be "moral agents"; that is, they are capable of acting autonomously, have preferences, and possess the ability to initiate actions to achieve goals. The principal right of all moral agents is the right to respectful treatment. This includes the right not to be killed (no matter how painlessly) because you cannot exercise your other rights if someone has deprived you of life.[54]

These arguments assume that no morally relevant differences exist between humans and the rest of the animal kingdom. But aren't such differences obvious? Most people think so. However, such differences are surprisingly difficult to demonstrate. As our scientific understanding of animals has grown over the previous decades, the continuities between humans and other animals appear to be stronger than previously believed. Let's examine some of the points most commonly raised in these debates.

How Different Are Humans and Other Animals?

Many people argue that, unlike people, nonhuman animals are incapable of feeling pain. However, evidence from three sources indicates that most animals are as capable of suffering as are humans.

First, research in comparative neuropsychology indicates that there are no significant structural differences between the nervous systems of humans and other animals.[55] Instead, the mechanisms of pain perception, including the sensory receptors in the skin, the neural pathways that convey pain messages to the central nervous system, and the brain structures that "register" pain, are common to most species.[56] This reflects our common evolutionary history. It is true that humans, compared with most other animals, have a large cerebral cortex—the part of the brain used for higher thought. But this difference is one of degree rather than kind. As Brian Kolb and Ian Whishaw, two neuropsychologists, point out:

> To many people, including many psychologists, both human neuroanatomy and human cognitive processes (i.e., thinking) fundamentally differ from those of animals. After all, humans talk, read, write, and do all sorts of things that no monkey or rat has ever done. It is our view that this line of reasoning is shortsighted and wrong. . . . There is no compelling evidence that there is a qualitative difference between the brains of humans and those of other mammals.[57]

Second, behavioral studies reveal that animals and humans react in similar ways to aversive stimuli such as electric shocks or burns; that is, they cry out and try to escape. Like humans, animals in pain also secrete adrenaline and reveal increases in blood pressure, heart rate, respiration, and general metabolic activity. However, when animals are given pain-killing drugs they do not exhibit these reactions. Similarly, if injured, both humans and animals will clutch a damaged limb and keep it still. And animals, like humans, learn to avoid behaviors that are physically punished. These common behaviors indicate that nonhuman animals do not like pain any more than humans do.[58]

Third, the theory of evolution holds that the experience of pain has survival value for a species in that it informs individuals that they are in danger (for example, when being attacked) and that they should escape as quickly as possible. Pain also teaches animals that aversive and potentially dangerous things, such as fire, should be avoided. Because the ability to suffer is adaptive, pain is likely to be experienced by all living things with highly developed nervous systems who have some degree of control over their environments and are capable of moving from one place to another.[59] This, of course, would include most animals and fish but would exclude all plants. (Plants have no nervous systems and so cannot experience pain. And because they cannot escape from danger, the ability to perceive pain confers no evolutionary advantage.) In addition, the fact that many species of plants evolve thorns, barbs, and needles as forms of protection is also informative, for they would only be effective against animals capable of feeling pain.

Many argue that humans are more intelligent than animals. Although this is certainly true, recent research reveals that animals are more intelligent than previously believed. Animals of many species are capable of making and using tools,[60] have elaborate communication systems, [61] live in complexly organized societies,[62] cooperate to achieve common goals, and help one another.[63] Furthermore, much of the behavior of animals is learned—not guided by instinct as was once thought. Most animals are capable of learning new skills and can even teach these to their offspring. Many people, for example, would be aware of recent studies in which rudimentary American sign language has been successfully taught to a variety of primates, including chimpanzees, gorillas, and orangutans. Chimpanzee mothers have been observed teaching many of these signs to their children.[64]

Some people argue that animals are incapable of making free choices. But animals do appear to show preferences for things and to act on the basis of plans and goals. Research on problem-solving in higher mammals, such as chimpanzees, indicates that they are capable of planning and carrying out complex sequences of activities to achieve a reward, such as food.[65] Indeed, one might ask, who is more goal-directed—the lioness who stalks her next meal or the man who treads the well-beaten path from the television to the refrigerator for his next beer?

Finally, some claim that humans have souls and animals do not. It is difficult to say whether animals—or humans for that matter—have souls. Many Eastern religions say that animals do;

Western religions say that they do not. Regardless of who is right, it would seem a poor justification for harming animals.

Implications

Few people subscribe to the morality that an action is permissible simply because one possesses the power to carry it out. As Mohandas Gandhi argued, the fact that we are more intelligent than animals and have power over them does not give us the right to exploit them. To the contrary, we are obligated to protect them.[66] For individuals who agree with these ethical arguments, vegetarianism is mandatory.

THE MOVEMENTS FOR SOCIAL JUSTICE AND PEACE

A belief in social progress has emerged at various times in history, for example, during the 18th century Enlightenment and during the Victorian era of humanitarian reform. Although World War I knocked the notion of social evolution on the head and ushered in an era of pessimism, the last few decades have seen a revitalization of the quest for a better society. This was manifested during the 1960s in the civil rights movement, in the 1970s in the feminist movement, and in the 1980s in the peace and antinuclear movements. Perhaps the desire for, and belief in, a better world is a reaction to the fact that things have become worse in the last few decades. Because the next war may be our last, people rightly feel that the quest for compassion, justice, and world peace is now more imperative than ever.

Many believe that the habit of eating meat has implications for how one relates to others. One frequently expressed notion is that of a link between meat-eating and cruelty, and correspondingly, between vegetarianism and compassion. The basic idea is that by treating animals cruelly or kindly, one comes to behave in a similar fashion toward people. For example, the philosopher Porphyry wrote, "He who abstains from anything animate . . . will be much more careful not to injure those of his own species. For he who loves the genus will not hate any species of animal."[67] More recently, the case was strongly stated by Philip Kepleau, founder of the Zen Center in New York:

> There is a causal relationship between the cruelty, torture, and death of human beings and the ongoing slaughter of millions of pigs, cows, fowl, and sheep. . . . How is it possible to swallow the carcasses of these slain creatures and not have hatred, aggression, and violence stimulated in oneself and others?[68]

Many prominent vegetarians have adopted their diet as part of a general philosophy of nonviolence, including Leo Tolstoy, Mohandas Gandhi, Dick Gregory, Scott Nearing, and Isaac Bashevis Singer. Vegetarians of this persuasion believe that world peace, if it is ever to be achieved, must be based on an attitude of nonviolence that encompasses animals as well as humans. Indeed, refraining from killing and eating animals may be a prerequisite for peace between nations. As Isaac Bashevis Singer stated:

> I personally believe that as long as human beings will go on shedding the blood of animals, there will never be any peace. There is only one little step from killing animals to creating gas chambers à la Hitler and concentration camps à la Stalin. . . . There will be no justice as long as man will stand with a knife or with a gun and destroy those who are weaker than he is.[69]

Of course, simply refraining from eating animals is unlikely, in and of itself, to lead to a more peaceful lifestyle. Adolf Hitler, for example, ate little meat; yet he can hardly be described as a peace-loving person. Rather, it is a belief in nonviolence that leads to an attitude of reverence for all forms of life—human as well as nonhuman. Killing an animal is seen by many as an act of violence. Consequently, by refusing to participate in the unnecessary killing of animals, these individuals make their everyday behavior consistent with a general principle of harmlessness. And, it is argued, by abandoning the slaughter of animals, society would teach and reinforce values of compassion and nonviolence—values that are necessary for the achievement of world peace.

Many people believe that the world will one day be vegetarian. This is partly because they are aware that vegetarianism will contribute in a practical way to the feeding of a hungry world. But more than this, people see vegetarianism as a higher form of society—the next stage of social evolution. As Henry David Thoreau stated:

> I have no doubt that it is part of the destiny of the human race, in its gradual improvement, to leave off eating animals, as surely as the savage tribes have left off eating each other when they come in contact with the more civilized.[70]

SUMMARY

As we noted earlier, contemporary vegetarians have been able to draw on a rich variety of movements, traditions, and bodies of knowledge for insight and motivation. The result of this convergence of forces has been an unprecedented wave of interest in vegetarianism in the West. This interest has been reflected in an increase in the number of organizations, restaurants, newsletters, magazines, books, cookbooks, and commercial food products for vegetarians. In the chapters that follow, we examine the experiences of individual vegetarians who have been shaped by, and in turn, have helped to shape, the social currents that have made vegetarianism a popular lifestyle in our times.

Chapter 2

Why Do People Become Vegetarians?

As we noted earlier, a variety of historical developments and social trends have made vegetarianism a growing and influential force today. But while it is one thing to understand something about these large-scale social movements, it is quite another to understand the experiences of particular individuals who live as vegetarians. In this chapter and the ones that follow, we turn to our interviews, questionnaires, and letters from vegetarians to describe what it is like to live as a herbivore in an omnivorous society. We begin by describing how we located people for our study.

LOCATING VEGETARIANS

At first we thought it would be difficult to find vegetarians. We knew, according to the Gallup poll referred to earlier, that a large and increasing number of Americans identify themselves as vegetarians. But how could we get in contact with them? And, more importantly, how could we persuade them to share their private beliefs and experiences with us?

We began by placing notices in newsletters of vegetarian organizations describing our project and asking people to write to us. Most of the newsletters we used are in the United States, but we also placed notices in English and Australian publications. In our request, we asked people to comment on a variety of topics: their reasons for rejecting meat, the implications of their diets for their physical and psychological well-being, the reactions of their friends and families, any problems they have had in being vegetarians, and any benefits they have experienced. We also asked parents to comment on the special problems they might have had in raising vegetarian children.

Given the amount of information asked for, we anticipated that few people would respond to our query. As it turned out, we quickly received 209 detailed accounts of people's experiences, many of which ran up to 10 pages or more in length. Another 61 people wrote and said they would be happy to answer specific questions. We sent these people a questionnaire to complete. As we discovered, many vegetarians are enthusiastic about discussing their diets; in many cases, respondents reported that no one had ever asked for their views on these topics before. After a short while our files reached the bursting point, and we had to start turning down requests to contribute to the project.

To supplement the types of information obtained from these "long-distance" contacts, we personally carried out in-depth interviews with 50 vegetarians living on the West Coast. These interviews were solicited through requests to local vegetarian clubs, notices on bulletin boards in natural food stores, ads in local papers, and word-of-mouth. Altogether, we collected information from 320 vegetarians.

The majority of our respondents (82%) live in the United States. In addition, 6 percent live in England, 5 percent live in Australia, 5 percent live in Canada, and 2 percent live elsewhere. The American respondents came from virtually every state in the Union, although the East and West Coasts are most strongly represented.

CHARACTERISTICS OF VEGETARIANS

The people described in this book hold a variety of occupations. Forty percent are in professional or managerial positions. Doctors, nurses, psychologists, dieticians, scientists, engineers, commercial artists, and company managers are examples of occupations represented in our sample. Nine percent of people in our study work in clerical or sales positions and 24 percent hold blue-collar jobs. Examples of these occupations include bank teller, secretary, laborer, mechanic, waitress, and taxi driver. In addition, 12 percent are homemakers, and 16 percent are students. Although the socioeconomic spread of our sample is broad, respondents with white-collar occupations clearly form the largest group.

Seventy-one percent of our respondents are women and only 29 percent are men. This gender imbalance reflects the fact that the majority of vegetarians are women—a finding consistent with earlier surveys. There are several possible reasons for this preponderance of women among the ranks of vegetarians. For one thing, women tend to be more sympathetic and compassionate than men, and hence, more likely to stop eating animals for ethical reasons. In addition, men are more likely than women to believe a number of myths about meat, for example, that meat is necessary to do hard work or to maintain one's virility.

The ages of people in our sample range from 11 to 90, with a median age of 35. Several children wrote to us because they felt it was important for young people's experiences to be included in our book. At the other end of the scale, many elderly vegetarians took time off from their usual activities, such as managing businesses, working for animal rights, jogging, bicycling, and hiking, to write to us.

In terms of diets, 34 percent of the people described in this book are lacto-ovo-vegetarians, 11 percent are lacto-vegetarians, 3 percent are ovo-vegetarians, 39 percent are vegans, 3 percent are natural hygienists, 1 percent practice macrobiotics, 1 percent are raw foodists or fruitarians, and 8 percent are semi-vegetarians. The length of time people have been vegetarian ranges from several months to 70 years, with a median of 8 years. The people in our study have been vegetarian, collectively, for a total of 3298 years—a substantial amount of experience for us to draw on for our study.

Is our sample representative of all vegetarians? There are

two ways of answering this question. On the one hand, people who volunteered to be in our study may differ in certain ways from those who did not volunteer. For example, ethical vegetarians and vegans, because they feel strongly about their diets, are more likely than other types of vegetarians to volunteer. In this sense, our group of vegetarians probably does not represent, in the correct proportions, all the various types of vegetarians who exist in the larger community. On the other hand, our sample is very broad in terms of geographical region, age, occupational background, type of diet, and length of time spent as a vegetarian. A wide variety of experiences and points of view are represented, and no major group of vegetarians has been omitted. Consequently, we are confident that the themes that emerge in this book provide an accurate and comprehensive picture of contemporary vegetarian lifestyles.

REASONS FOR BECOMING A VEGETARIAN

One of the first things people ask when they encounter a vegetarian is, "Why don't you eat meat?" We used this fundamental question as the starting point for our own interviews. In sorting through people's responses, we identified 11 general motives for becoming vegetarian. These motives, and the percentage of people who expressed them, are: a concern over animal suffering or a belief in animal rights (67%), a desire to promote personal health (38%), religious beliefs or a wish to live a more spiritual life (17%), a dislike of meat or a sensitivity to aesthetics (12%), the pursuit of personal growth (7%), a concern about world hunger (5%), a desire for a nonviolent lifestyle (5%), an interest in improving the environment (5%), a belief that meat-eating is unnatural for humans (4%), the high cost of meat (3%), and social conformity (1%). A small number of people (1%) held idiosyncratic motives that did not fit into these categories. In addition, 1 percent of people claimed to have had no particular reason for becoming vegetarian; they just did it.

The above percentages add up to more than 100 because many people expressed more than one motive. In our sample,

43 percent of people had a single reason for becoming vegetarian and 57 percent expressed multiple reasons. This tells us that the majority of people are "complex" vegetarians who see a variety of advantages in a meatless diet. As it turns out, "single issue" vegetarians were mainly animal rights supporters. For these people, a concern with animal ethics is a sufficient reason for rejecting the eating of flesh.

Animal Ethics

A concern with animal ethics is the most frequently mentioned reason for becoming vegetarian. (We cannot, however, conclude that this is the most common reason held by vegetarians in general—only by the vegetarians in our sample.) Ethical vegetarians express their concern in two major ways: an emotional reaction to animal suffering, and a belief in the principle that animals have fundamental rights.

People who express concern over the suffering of animals usually refer to conditions on factory farms. Earlier, we described the modern meat industry's harsh treatment of animals. This discovery comes as a shock to many people and upsets them greatly. Some literally give up meat on the spot after learning of the conditions experienced by many farm animals. Not surprisingly, these people typically describe their "conversion" in emotional terms. Some say that their consciences will never allow them to eat meat again.

> I'd always blindly accepted the myth that animals are treated well until they are humanely killed for man's benefit. Once my eyes were opened to the widespread sadism and torture inflicted upon farm animals, I could never eat another creature again.

> After discovering the reality of the plight of animals used for food, I stopped all consumption. The fact that animals live in "concentration camps" and go through needless and endless mutilation, torture, and suffering for man's depraved greed and evil was my initiation into the world of eating nonanimals.

> I felt in my heart, mind, and soul that eating an animal was

> totally insane, inhumane, and I knew it was wrong. My conscience told me so.

Other people are motivated less by an emotional concern with animal suffering and more by an abstract conviction that animals, along with humans, should be accorded certain rights. They feel that, regardless of whether or not suffering is involved, killing and eating animals is a violation of the animal's most basic right: the right to life. Some people extend their moral philosophy mainly to mammals; others feel that all forms of life have certain rights. These people typically rely less on appeals to emotion than on logical argument to make their point.

> I believe that pigs and cows and goats are sentient beings with feelings and intelligence enough to justify that we not kill them to eat. Pigs are at least as intelligent as dogs and the American public is opposed to eating dogs. But intelligent or not, they do have feelings of fear and are capable of suffering.

> The animals we eat are capable of experiencing pleasure and pain. Now, the amount of benefit that we gain from eating animals is quite small compared with the amount of suffering animals go through in being slaughtered. Therefore, in all fairness, the rights of animals to live and enjoy their lives must take precedence over our "right" to eat whatever we desire.

Earlier we noted that people motivated by a belief in animal rights often found this single motive to be sufficient to lead to a commitment to vegetarianism, with no other supporting motives being necessary. The following quote from Derrick,* a systems programmer, is a good example of this perspective:

> I did it, not in order to improve my health, not for religious reasons (East or West), not to avoid the high cost of meat, not to contribute to a more rational food distribution around the world or to preserve the Brazilian rain forests, but because I recognized that I have no right to participate in animal slavery and animal killing, no matter how good the taste of meat.

*Throughout the book, the names of respondents have been changed to protect their anonymity.

Some individuals who view themselves as animal lovers become aware of the inconsistency between caring for animals and eating them. Many who have this experience feel that they are hypocrites. The realization that they are acting in violation of their own values provides a sufficient motivation for these people to change their behavior. Ben, an accountant, put it this way:

> I did it because I just started thinking about where the meat came from. I realized I was a hypocrite, as a supposed animal lover. If I really care about animals, how can I possibly promote an industry based on such terrible cruelty to animals?

Most people become aware of these issues through contact with the animal welfare movement, either through reading animal rights literature or through direct contact with a member of an animal rights organization. Most ethical vegetarians prefer not to be actively involved in the movement, but nevertheless feel that refraining from eating meat is an important contribution they can make in their own lives. Other people decide to join an animal rights organization and adopt vegetarianism at the same time, as part of an overall change in lifestyle. In contrast, some people are active in the animal rights movement for years before they finally make a commitment to stop eating flesh. For example, Robyn, an interior designer, said:

> My adoption of a vegetarian diet came as a direct result of my belated but wholehearted interest in the plight of animals and the evils of speciesism. For many years the issues of human cruelty to animals gnawed at the edges of my consciousness. Finally, as the movement for animal rights became more vocal, awareness penetrated.

Although many ethical vegetarians are influenced by the animal rights movement, others come to the conclusion that eating animals is wrong on their own. In some cases, for a period of time, a person thinks that he or she is the only person in the world who doesn't eat animals for moral reasons. For these individuals, discovering that other ethical vegetarians exist comes as a surprise—and a relief.

A few people are led to ethical vegetarianism through working with animals. For example, Roger's training as an experimental psychologist led to the realization that animals, like humans, are capable of experiencing pain:

> My motivation for vegetarian eating arose chiefly from a belief that animals should not be killed for trivial purposes. I have always had pet cats or dogs. My observations of these animal friends and my studies in psychology convinced me that there is a continuity in the cognitive and emotional processes between humans and nonhuman animals, and that killing animals for food is invariably accompanied by pain and terror for the animals. It is easy to imagine this as cruelty if one's pet cat or dog were being slaughtered. I concluded that it is no less cruel just because the animal is unnamed or unknown to one, or is killed in the secluded confines of a slaughterhouse.

The many comments quoted above illustrate the power of ethical motives. Once people are convinced that killing and eating animals is ethically wrong, their consciences, and their need to think of themselves as responsible people, require that they live as vegetarians. It is an orientation to one's diet that is relatively demanding. Because refraining from meat is a moral imperative, lapses generate feelings of guilt and remorse. Consequently, ethical vegetarians are less likely than those motivated by other concerns to revert back to meat-eating, either temporarily or permanently.

Health

A concern over health is another major reason for abstaining from meat. Health vegetarians can be divided into two groups: those who are primarily concerned with food additives, and those who are primarily concerned with the role of meat and animal fat in various degenerative diseases.

Those in the first group adopt a vegetarian diet, not so much because of the meat itself, but because of the antibiotics, growth hormones, and stimulants given to farm animals, as well as the chemicals used to treat and preserve meats. People concerned about the additives found in meat typically try to avoid all processed foods that contain artificial ingredients and preservatives.

> I became a vegetarian for health reasons. All the antibiotics and the way they raise and kill animals is unhealthy. I feel that we are exposed to enough risks and we should really try to eliminate the ones that we can.

> I didn't want to eat meat that was pumped up with chemicals and dyes. My whole diet excludes packaged or processed foods with preservatives.

The second, and larger, group of health vegetarians are those concerned about the implications of a diet containing high levels of animal fat for heart disease, cancer, and other health disorders. A number of people in this group work in the medical professions. As such, they are familiar with the recent medical literature linking diet to a variety of degenerative diseases. For example, Augusta, a medical doctor, told us:

> Our family became vegetarians because of health reasons. My husband and I, both physicians, had family histories that were not very favorable to good health and long length of life—such as diabetes, hypertension, cancer, and heart disease. All of these are known to be diet related, and we had known since we were in medical school that a vegetarian diet was the most favorable diet for any of these diseases.

Martin, a physician, told us about his experiences in prescribing a vegan diet for a range of medical problems:

> I utilize nutritional counseling as a keystone of my medical practice. I have been vegan for five years and have been impressed and often amazed at the beneficial effects of an animal-free diet upon human health. Many, if not most, degenerative diseases in our society today, such as heart attacks, strokes, diabetes, cancer, arthritis, and many allergies, can be prevented and often greatly improved by a diet free of animal fat and dairy products. My clinical practice has provided me with many instances of dramatic beneficial changes in these conditions through vegan nutrition. The many subsequent corroborating articles in the medical

> literature have only confirmed my beliefs that vegan nutrition holds the key to human health in the 20th century and beyond.

Some health vegetarians are completely unaware of the medical literature showing a correlation between meat-centered diets and various diseases. Instead, they discover through personal experience that they feel better and are generally healthier when not eating meat. These people typically start off adopting a vegetarian diet for a period of time as an experiment; later, when they find they like the outcome, their commitment to vegetarianism is established. Roy was traveling around the country with "no destination and a pocketful of money" when he had the following experiences:

> I started paying attention to how I felt after eating certain types of food. I noticed that when I ate meat, my body felt heavy and dull, and that when I ate vegetarian meals, my body usually felt good. Later I did a lot of reading on nutrition, and I experimented with different types of diets. I decided that I was definitely healthier as a vegetarian.

The notion that a meatless diet is health-promoting is consistent with the medical research we reviewed earlier. It is also supported by the many personal accounts we heard from health vegetarians. Some told us that they had suffered from health problems for years and had turned to vegetarianism as a way of dealing with them. We describe some of these cases in detail later when we discuss the personal implications of a meatless diet. It is worth pointing out here, however, that for these people, a change in diet (often accompanied by other changes in lifestyle, such as increased exercise) resulted in major and dramatic improvements in health, and this became a powerful motive for their continuing to live as vegetarians.

Religion

Religious beliefs, or a desire to live a more spiritual life, constitute another important motive for abstaining from flesh. Religious vegetarians can be divided into three groups. First, some people belong to religious groups in which vegetarianism is either required (such as the International Society for Krishna Consciousness) or strongly recommended (such as the Seventh-Day Adventists). In most cases, these people give up flesh when they convert to their new faith. Second, some people belong to religions that do not have a strong vegetarian tradition, such as Catholicism or Judaism. Nevertheless, these people feel that a meatless diet is consistent with the ethical teachings of their religions. Third, some people do not belong to a formal organized religion, but believe that a meatless diet allows them to live a more spiritual existence.

Among religions that advocate vegetarianism, those emanating from India are the most common. As we discussed earlier, many Eastern religions discourage the eating of meat because it is believed that animals, as well as humans, have souls. Because of this, killing and eating animals incurs a moral debt that a person must one day repay. We spoke with several members of the International Society for Krishna Consciousness who explained their personal reasons for being vegetarians. Some worried about the negative consequences of eating animals, whereas others felt that a vegetarian diet makes one more receptive to spiritual values.

> When I joined the Hare Krishna movement I learned about the violent slaughter of animals and the karmic effects of eating meat. The reason for the diet is to lessen the karma, so you can get out of this cycle of death and rebirth.

> I became a Hare Krishna devotee and, of course, the Vedic Scriptures are insistent about being a vegetarian. Giving up the eating of meat helps clear the mind and open the heart to religious ideas.

We also spoke with several members of the Kirpal Light Satsang in San Diego—another religious group with its roots in India—who explained the connection between their religious beliefs and their diets. Richard told us:

> Our spiritual master, Thakar Singh, says that for spiritual meditation, the particles of meat inhibit the soul from being

attuned to the inner sound current. Eating a more subtle diet, with finer particles, helps the process.

Followers of Sri Chinmoy—a religious teacher from India—are also vegetarian. Sujantra, a member of the Sri Chinmoy group in San Diego, explained his reasons for not eating meat:

> I've found that the vibrations of food affect my nerves on a very subtle level. It aids your meditation to eat foods that have a milder vibration, like fruits and vegetables, and to stay away from foods like meat. In order to meditate and to pray, you don't have to be vegetarian. And because someone is a vegetarian doesn't mean that they are any more spiritual than anyone else. Yet, being a vegetarian can enhance your meditation because of the peaceful vibration in the food.

As noted above, Western religions are also represented among the ranks of religious vegetarians. Several people in our sample were Seventh-Day Adventists—a religious group with a strong vegetarian tradition. Seventh-Day Adventists believe that meat, particularly meat produced by factory farm methods, is often tainted with disease and is generally unhealthy. Because Christians should maintain good health in order to do God's work, eating meat is frowned upon by the church. Tom, a pastor in the Seventh-Day Adventist Church, explained his views on eating flesh. As he pointed out, good reasons can be found in the Bible to justify a vegetarian diet.

> Seventh-Day Adventists get their perspective from the Bible. In the beginning, when God created people, he created them vegetarian. There would be no death, and consequently, there would be no death of animals, so there would be no meat. If you read genealogies up to the flood, you will find that people lived to be seven, eight, nine hundred years old. Right after the flood, you will find that when man was permitted to eat meat, his life expectancy decreased rapidly to three score and ten. It almost looks as if there was a direct relationship between the two. We recognize that there are hundreds of diseases that an animal can have, and many of those can be communicated to humans . . . . The devil has a three-pronged attack. He's got a

> poor theology, which will destroy your spiritual life. He also has things that will destroy your mind. And then he has things that will destroy your body. Meat is one of them. So we encourage people to be vegetarian.

Mormons are not allowed to drink alcohol or to smoke. Steve, a Mormon, believed that his religion also required him to be a vegetarian. As he explained to us:

> I first gave up meat because our religion asks us to eat meat only if we need to sustain ourselves. In the Doctrines and Covenants—which the Mormons would consider to be a revelation from Jesus Christ through Joseph Smith—it says that it is pleasing to the Lord to eat meat only in times of cold winter or famine. I interpret that to mean that we should eat meat only to sustain ourselves when we can't get other food.

However, Steve admitted that few people in his church agree with his interpretation of this particular passage. Although many Mormons eat meat in moderation, relatively few are true vegetarians.

Some Christians do not belong to a church or sect that formally encourages vegetarianism. Nevertheless, many find a meatless diet to be consistent with their own understanding of the Bible and Christ's teachings. Some believe that the treatment of animals in modern factory farms contradicts the Christian values of kindness and compassion. Others feel that killing and eating animals is a violation of the general injunction not to kill unnecessarily. As some commented:

> God declared, straight from the Bible, any pork consumption is a sin. He also informed us as to what He allowed us to eat. God intended animal consumption, but never any suffering to any life that He created. Man has decided to make a mockery of God's commandments. The end result: the hideous suffering of innocent, helpless, beautiful creatures.

> I always quote the Ten Commandments: Thou shalt not kill. It doesn't say kill what. It just says thou shalt not kill. But those people who enjoy meat change the rules around to say that God didn't mean animals—only people.

Finally, as noted above, some religious vegetarians do not belong to any particular religion—East or West—or adhere to any particular doctrine. Nevertheless, they feel that being vegetarian allows them to achieve a more spiritual life than would otherwise be possible. To some, the killing of animals for food—an act of violence—is incompatible with higher spiritual ideals. Others believe that eating meat stimulates base, carnal desires.

> I wanted to be spiritually enlightened and I didn't think that eating animal foods was a part of that enlightenment. I became vegetarian to be healthier, saner, lighter, and closer to God.
>
> I think I was led by God to become more aware of my love for animals in order to improve my spirituality. Humans and animals are all God's creatures, and if we are to evolve, we must be in tune with our fellow spirits. I believe animals are beings and have souls or spirits. We have a moral duty to treat animals as we would like to be treated ourselves.

All in all, the particular beliefs of religious vegetarians are diverse, with some drawing their inspiration primarily from Eastern religions and others adhering more to Western religions. But in spite of their diversity of views, they all share a belief that being a vegetarian is good for the soul and brings one closer to God.

Aesthetics

Another group of vegetarians give up flesh for "aesthetic" reasons; that is, they feel that meat is unappealing, unappetizing, or downright repulsive. Many people in this group say they avoid flesh because they do not like its flavor or texture. In some cases, people have felt this way since childhood, and consequently, have never been big meat eaters. For these people, becoming vegetarian is simply a matter of following their natural preferences. As John, a produce manager in a food store, claimed:

> Meat does not appeal to me sufficiently for me to go through the bother of eating it. I've never been drawn to

> meat. I have never looked up and seen a rabbit or any other animal and salivated and thought that was what I wanted to eat. It has always been fruit that I found to be appealing, even as a child.

In other cases, people develop an aversion to animal flesh later in life. Sometimes this change is linked to a specific experience, such as visiting a slaughterhouse. More often, a dislike of meat is linked to a gradually evolving awareness of what meat really is. People who think clearly about where the steaks on their plates come from cannot escape the fact that meat is nothing more than the muscle tissue, fat, veins, and blood of a dead animal. Once people fully realize what they are eating, many find it impossible to dine on meat with a hearty appetite. For these individuals, vegetarianism is the next step.

> The concept of eating animals began more and more to revolt me, regardless of how humanely the animal was raised. One day I finally said, "I don't want to eat cows anymore. It's an animal and it's disgusting."

> Eating the carcass of an animal is gross: the blood, the bones, the muscle tissue. If you think about it, it's enough to make you throw up.

On the positive side, some people enjoy being vegetarian because vegetarian food is delicious and tastes better than meat. As Sharon put it, "Part of what sold me was how delicious vegetarian cuisine actually is." Often these people start off, like many others, expecting meatless meals to be tasteless and boring. A few encounters with well-prepared vegetarian food at restaurants or friends' homes, however, convince them that they can derive considerable gastronomic pleasure living as vegetarians.

Personal Growth

Personal growth vegetarians place their primary emphasis on self-development. They recognize that abstaining from animal flesh confers many benefits, including improvements in health, spirituality, and a sense of moral purpose. The particular benefits themselves, however, are less important than the fact that vegetarianism helps them to grow and to achieve their full potential. As George, a physics graduate student, said, "I want to be the best that I can be, so I decided that I should be vegetarian."

Many people in this group spend years trying out different philosophies, religions, and therapies. Some describe themselves as "searchers" or "seekers." In most cases, vegetarianism is adopted as one component of a larger and continuing process of self-growth. For a few, vegetarianism occupies a central role as the key element in their personal development. The following are examples of a personal growth perspective:

> Over the past three years, I've been changing my whole lifestyle. Vegetarianism was just one of many issues I'd been dealing with. It is related to the desire to find a simpler, cleaner, saner, and more compassionate way of life. My reasons were spiritual, physical, and emotional. It was my time to become a vegetarian. It was the next natural progression for me. It didn't even involve any physical thought or effort. The move was wholly intuitive and necessary.

> I saw vegan people and they were the nicest, kindest, happiest, healthiest, and most loving people I have met. I knew it was a way to spiritual enlightenment and purity. I'm a searcher for everything good and it is a higher way.

In contrast to an emphasis on positive growth, a few adopt a vegetarian diet as a way of correcting some perceived fault in their characters. These people might be described as "vegetarian Puritans." For example, Mark stopped eating meat to refine his sexual urges and make them less "bestial." Another individual felt that meat-eating was a form of gluttony: a self-indulgent and unnecessary gratification of the senses. As such, meat-eating was a weakness to be overcome:

> I had sorrow and suffering due to my gluttony. I was suffering from psychic pain caused by over-nutrition. I used to be addicted to meat excesses as a true sensualist. So, in order to subordinate my appetite to my weak will power, I decided to adopt complete vegetarianism.

World Hunger

Some people become vegetarian because they see meat consumption in the West as being partly responsible for world hunger. These individuals are aware of the wastefulness of livestock production as a source of food. As we pointed out earlier, a larger number of people can be supported by using a given area of land to grow crops directly for human consumption than by using the land to grow crops to feed livestock.

> During college, I interned at the United Nations where I did some research on hunger and food issues. I became aware of the wasteful inequities involved in meat production, and how a large portion of the world goes to bed hungry each night because of our food choices.

> I was very concerned with the suffering of others on a world-wide level and felt that my eating of meat contributed to the problems, so I had to stop. Feeding food that people can eat, such as grains and beans, to animals for slaughter is crazy when there are so many people starving.

These individuals believe that becoming vegetarian is one small but necessary step in decreasing the demand for meat in the West, and hence, in the eventual freeing of land for producing crops that could be used to feed the poor. Even this small act gives people a sense that they have done something useful and positive. As Roberta said, "I figured we can't change the world, but I can contribute a little bit toward eliminating world hunger."

For many, abstaining from meat is a symbolic gesture of solidarity with hungry people around the world. At the same time, it also represents a rejection of the wasteful practices, and the mixed-up values, of our own society.

> I am keenly aware of the wasteful indulgent practices of America. Giving up meat seemed like a definite step we were able to make now to put us in solidarity with the millions who live on a meatless diet by necessity. The exploitation of other countries for our own luxury infuriates me.

Millie and Bob are examples of vegetarians who are concerned about world hunger. Together, they operate a farm in Maine designed to serve as a model of self-sufficiency in food production. They are also involved in investigating new techniques of forestry and energy production that are environmentally sound. As they told us, "We became vegetarians because of land use. It's wasteful of land to be meat and animal product eaters. Becoming farmers has made it all much more understandable."

Nonviolence

Many vegetarians do not distinguish between the killing of animals and the killing of humans. Accordingly, they see a link between their diets and issues of peace and nonviolence. For some, this link is a very personal one, whereas for others it has society-wide implications.

At the personal level, some vegetarians adopt a philosophy of harmlessness toward all living things. For these people, to eat meat is to participate in a deplorable act of violence—even murder. They believe that as vegetarians, they are eliminating an unwanted and unnecessary source of violence from their lives.

> I decided that I did not want to harm or kill anything. I wanted my conscience to be clear of that kind of guilt. We do not have the right to inflict violence on anything, including animals.
>
> As long as we tolerate the widespread slaughter of other species, it puts a hardness in us. Every time we eat meat, we perpetuate that, if only on an unconscious level. Violence begins on your dinner table.

On a broader level, rejecting all forms of violence in one's own life may have a beneficial effect on the larger society. Some individuals believe that adopting a nonviolent vegetarian diet is a small but positive step for world peace. Often, these people work or have worked in the peace movement. Over time, they have come to feel that it is hypocritical to work for world peace and, at the same time, dine on the bodies of slaughtered animals. Many believe that by living as vegetarians, they set a positive example of nonviolence for others and become more effective in advocating the cause of peace. To be a true pacifist, some argue, one must be a vegetarian. Marilyn, a masseuse, put it this way:

> It's something like a nonviolence pledge. I wanted to take on a nonviolent lifestyle, and I figured that to get rid of violence in the world you can begin with what you're eating.

The Environment

As pointed out earlier, some people come to vegetarianism via the environmental movement. These "environmental vegetarians" are sometimes conservationists directly involved in preserving our wildlife. Some are members of Greenpeace or other activist environmental groups. For these people, the main reason for adopting a vegetarian diet is to minimize the destructive effects of livestock production on our soil, water, forests, and wildlife. As Dean, a commercial artist, wrote:

> My concern for the environment is what keeps me going. I'm saying "No" to the fast food hamburger chains' destruction of rainforest for grazing land, "No" to overgrazing the continent of Africa and the resulting starvation of millions, and "No" to the human aggression toward all living creatures.

Hope and her husband are examples of vegetarians who are concerned about conservation. Together, they operate a wildlife refuge in New Jersey. She explained to us how her efforts to preserve wildlife and her concern over the impact of hunting led her to become a vegetarian:

> We settled in southern New Jersey where we soon became aware of how development was ruining land and wildlife. We bought land for a wildlife refuge, and it was while patrolling our posted land that something happened to change our lives. One day I was talking with a hunter at our

> border. He knew our stand against killing and asked, "You eat meat, don't you?" When I said "Yes," he smiled and said, "A deer is just a cow. A quail is just a chicken. What's the difference?" As I walked home through the woods I pondered his question and had to admit that I was a hypocrite. I have never eaten meat since that day 25 years ago.

A Natural Way of Life

Some vegetarians believe that humans are designed to be plant-eaters and, correspondingly, that meat-eating is unnatural for our species. As supporting evidence, they point out that our physical makeup is more akin to that of herbivores than to carnivores. For example, carnivores, unlike humans, have sharp teeth for cutting through skin and bone; humans, like herbivores, have broad molars designed to grind plant foods. Carnivores, unlike humans, can run fast and have sharp claws for catching their prey; humans, on the other hand, are incapable of outrunning and catching an animal such as a deer or rabbit. And carnivores, unlike humans, have strong digestive acids and short intestines to excrete decaying animal matter quickly. Humans, like herbivores, have weak digestive acids and long intestines which are necessary for the slow digestion of plant foods. Many vegetarians believe that humans became "sidetracked" from their original diet.

Most "natural vegetarians" try to simplify their lives. They avoid accumulating material objects, recycle wastes when possible, and minimize their consumption of energy from fossil fuels. They prefer to spend their leisure time outdoors in rural areas and avoid the nightlife available in big cities. To them, vegetarianism is another change they have made on the way toward a simpler, more harmonious way of life.

John, who works at a food store, is a vegetarian because it is "more natural" than eating meat. He publishes his own natural foods newsletter, has few possessions, dresses simply, and spends as much time outdoors as possible. John told us that he could tell "instinctively" that meat was not well-suited for his body:

> Through meditation, I became more in touch with my instincts and more in tune with what my body wanted and what flesh was. It was actually the taking of a life and that was a violent thing. That didn't feel right within me as a human being.

Jack, who works in a food cooperative, says that his ideal world is one in which all things are left as untouched as possible. As he says, "I like things in their natural order, the way the universe intended." Jack, and others like him, feel that humans should not try to dominate and change the natural world, and that our present attitudes and behavior are likely to result in an ecological disaster. To Jack, nothing is more unnatural than keeping animals in captivity in modern factory farms. Not only are their meat and milk unsuited for human consumption, but keeping animals penned up and unable to roam freely is a violation of their natural inclinations.

Economics

For a few people, the initial reasons for giving up meat have less to do with their beliefs and values and more to do with harsh economic realities. Meat is a relatively expensive food item. Because of this, some people have their first encounter with vegetarianism during a period of poverty when they cannot afford to buy meat.

> Originally, it was for financial reasons. I had just been divorced and had very little money. I realized it was a lot cheaper not to buy meat. I would still have things like spaghetti sauce but without the meat.
>
> I was very poor living in the Rocky Mountains in a log cabin. I had next to nothing and I was literally living on $5 a month. I bought beans and rice, potatoes, and oatmeal.

In these cases, people soon discover other benefits of a meatless diet and continue to live as vegetarians after their financial situations improve.

Social Conformity

A few people stop eating meat primarily for social reasons. This typically occurs because they are living with people who are vegetarian. Under these circumstances, it is easier, and more fun, to become vegetarian as well. In one case, this came about when the person was living for a period of time with a family of vegetarians. She discovered that she enjoyed the diet and decided to stick to it when she later moved out. Another person adopted the diet during his college days after his roommates all gave up eating meat. Although relatively rare in our sample, as vegetarianism becomes more widespread, the number of people who give up eating meat for primarily social reasons will undoubtedly increase.

Other Motives

A small number of people have motives for giving up flesh that are idiosyncratic and difficult to classify. For example, one person became vegetarian for a change of pace:

> The basic reason for changing my diet was boredom. I was just really tired of my diet and wanted a change. The more I learned, and the more involved I got, the more I liked it. It was fun and a new learning experience.

One person took it on as a challenge, just to see if she could do it:

> Really, I did it just for the challenge of it. Whenever you challenge yourself—like fasting for a couple of days—you are also challenging yourself mentally. That was also part of the reason—to see how long I could do it.

For another person, vegetarianism was a way of setting herself apart from a society with which she largely disagreed:

> When I grew up and left school at 16, I looked around the world and realized what a wicked place it was and how dishonest, cruel, and underhanded most people were. I embraced vegetarianism eagerly but not for altruistic reasons. I wanted to be different because I did not want to be

> party to the ways of the world with its cruelties, stupid religions, and so on. By becoming vegetarian, I would be seen to be different in no uncertain manner.

A couple of people said they had no particular reason for becoming vegetarian; it just seemed like a good idea at the time. Clearly, these people are casual in their approach to life. In contrast, Jim had a complex philosophical position worked out:

> The primary reason was, and is, the desire not to be a predator. I figured that as long as my ultimate identity and purpose—as well as the true nature of this place—was unknown, I would be philosophically dishonest in killing animals just to maintain my own presence in this possibly meaningless parade of life and death. This does not imply that I assume it is wrong to kill animals and eat them. It seems that Whoever created this ecosystem in which we find ourselves designed some animals to eat other animals. We are fully a part of this system, but we have the option of choosing to go with either the consumer–consumee battle for survival, or to take a more mellow route. Either is legitimate. I believe those people who go hunting for deer or birds, or go fishing, and then eat what they kill are not doing anything wrong. But I want to take a different course.

OVERVIEW OF MOTIVES

Vegetarians hold a variety of diverse reasons for abstaining from meat. Overall, however, these motives can be divided into two broad groups: those that reflect ethical–social considerations (animal ethics, the environment, world hunger, and nonviolence) and those that reflect personal benefits (health, spirituality, aesthetics, personal growth, economics, a natural lifestyle, and social conformity). Classifying responses on this basis, 38 percent of the people in our sample are purely ethical–social vegetarians, 19 percent are personal benefit vegetarians, and 43 percent combine elements of both perspectives. This suggests that it is common to blend altruistic motives with self-gain motives in one's rationale for not eating flesh. Clearly, many people see vegetarianism as having benefits both for the self and for others.

CHANGES IN MOTIVES OVER TIME

The original reasons that people have for giving up meat may not be the same reasons they hold for continuing to live as vegetarians. To explore this issue, we asked people if their reasons for being vegetarian had changed in any way since they first stopped eating flesh. As it turns out, most people's reasons do change over time.

The most common pattern is for people to begin with a single motive and later to become aware and accepting of other reasons. Once people stop eating meat, for whatever motive, curiosity leads them to seek out information on other aspects of vegetarianism. In addition, questions and criticisms from meat-eaters lead many vegetarians to become better informed about the issues involved. As they do this, they discover new reasons for abstaining from meat; for many, these new reasons become more compelling than the original ones.

Some people start off for reasons of health or other personal benefits and later come to appreciate the ethical and social implications of what they are doing.

> I originally gave up animal foods for health and nutritional reasons. But the longer I remain vegan, the more I'm seeing that the eating of animals and animal by-products is morally wrong as well.
>
> I became vegetarian as a New Year's resolution. Three months later I attended an animal rights meeting and I walked out a vegan. My previous health reasons for abstaining from animal flesh quickly turned into a total, new ethical consideration of my diet and lifestyle.

As the above quotations suggest, early experimentation with a meatless diet can later grow into a deep and personal commitment. This level of commitment is often unanticipated by the novice vegetarian.

In other cases, people who originally become vegetarian out of a concern for animals or other social issues discover that personal health benefits are also important reasons for continuing a fleshless diet.

> My first reason was simply compassion for animals. But since my original revelations, my reasons have expanded and grown. Most meat is full of hormones, pesticide residues, large amounts of fat, and little dietary fiber. So health reasons have also come into play.

> I became a lacto-vegetarian strictly for moral and ethical reasons. I truthfully was unaware of the health problems involved in meat-eating until long after I had launched into vegetarianism. I had given no thought to the chemicals applied to animals which soak through their skin or the chemicals added to their feed to make them fat. Now I wonder how anyone can eat meat regardless of how they feel about animals. To me, meat is the unhealthiest food that can go into the body.

When people adopt new reasons, they are twice as likely to change from a concern with personal benefits to a concern with ethical–social issues as they are to do the reverse. This suggests a natural progression for people who originally stop eating meat for their own self-interest later to come to appreciate the larger ethical and social implications of their actions. In contrast, those who originally become vegetarian for altruistic reasons are less likely to explore, or acknowledge, the beneficial side effects for themselves. Perhaps this is because people with strong ethical motives tend to be less concerned with personal gain than others are. Alternatively, it may be that ethical vegetarians feel that explicitly accepting the personal benefits of a meatless diet might compromise the integrity and purity of their stand.

Another common pattern is for people not to change their initial reasons, but to become more certain of their beliefs and stronger in their convictions over time.

> I am only more convinced that my decision was sensible and right. As I learn more about factory/intensive farming conditions, my abhorrence of eating animal flesh becomes more acute.

> Over the years, I have become more and more committed to my lifestyle. My life is guided by a philosophy of compassion and reverence for life. I increasingly see the interconnections between that philosophy and a healthy, nonviolent, well-fed, ecologically sound world.

A few long-term vegetarians become so certain of their beliefs, and so committed to their lifestyles, that they rarely think about it anymore. It appears that the motives of these people are taken for granted and largely unconscious. As Ricky, a vegetarian of 15 years, said:

> Over the years, I've claimed every reason you can think of. I've been a spiritual vegetarian, a nonviolence vegetarian, an economic vegetarian, and a health vegetarian—all at one time or another. Now, it is so ingrained it is just the way it is.

VIEWS OF OTHER VEGETARIANS

Earlier, we noted that the majority of people embrace a variety of reasons for avoiding meat. Nevertheless, some emphasize one motive more than the others. We wondered if there might be cleavages—even a degree of hostility—between vegetarians from "opposing camps," such as health vegetarians versus ethical vegetarians. For this reason, we asked people about their views of vegetarians motivated by reasons different from their own.

We found little overt hostility. Instead, most people adopt an attitude of live and let live. But, there are some disagreements. Some vegetarians motivated by health or personal growth are mildly critical of ethical vegetarians. For example, one person on a macrobiotic diet had this to say about vegetarians concerned only about the welfare of animals:

> Some vegetarians are worried about killing animals, but this is basically a sentimental reason. We're all doing the same work, looking for a more humane way of life. But macrobiotics takes it one step further—out of the sentimental level to the intellectual level.

A few feel that ethical vegetarians—particularly animal rights activists—are too extreme. In contrast, they see themselves as having a more reasonable, moderate point of view.

> My reasons are mostly health[-related]. I'm not fanatical like some are about not wearing leather or buying fur coats.

> I don't want to be responsible for the killing of animals, but death is a part of life. A human being's survival is important. In situations where people need meat for health, I'm not opposed to killing animals.

> I don't think too much about the slaughtering of animals. My sorrow is more with children starving in the Third World than with the odd cow.

On the other hand, some ethical vegetarians are critical of people who abstain from flesh for purely health reasons. Some complain about "health food nuts" who take their diets too seriously. Others feel that health vegetarians do not show enough compassion for animals.

> Those who are in it for health reasons are real hypochondriacs and are always worried about their health or are stuck on themselves. They have this attitude that they're perfect, they're better than everybody else—high and mighty.

> It is very difficult for me to understand people who become vegetarians for health reasons only and have no feelings for the health of the animals. I feel they are selfish and narrow in their focus.

Another complaint sometimes voiced by ethical vegetarians about health vegetarians is that they lack true conviction. These people feel that those motivated by health concerns can easily go back to their old meat-eating habits if it is convenient or if they feel like a change of pace. Ethical vegetarians, on the other hand, cannot return to flesh-eating because this would violate a fundamental moral imperative. Alessandra, a writer, put it this way:

> Health vegetarians often seem to be fighting temptation, or slipping and feeling guilty. Because of my philosophy, I

> have no temptation; eating animals is simply not a possibility. If health conscious people could develop an animal rights philosophy, they'd have it made.

Ethical vegetarians do not direct all of their flak at health vegetarians; a few are also critical of those who abstain from flesh mainly to pursue spiritual interests. They feel that many spiritual vegetarians are out of touch with reality and as one person put it, "too far off the planet." Another individual said:

> The people who are into meditation and yoga take off on it a bit too much and a lot of them are floating around and are not on the earth. The animal rights people are a lot more like everyone else, except we don't eat meat.

Differences exist not only between vegetarians who hold different motives, but also between vegetarians who share the same motive. For example, some health vegetarians take exception to the diets of some of their peers. One person on a macrobiotic diet had this to say about lacto-ovo-vegetarians:

> I've seen many people who've gone on many different vegetarian diets and still come down with nutritional imbalances. Vegetarianism alone is not enough to guarantee health and personal development.

This person, of course, feels that macrobiotics represents the pinnacle of the vegetarian lifestyle. On the other hand, a lacto-ovo-vegetarian had this to say about macrobiotics:

> I got into macrobiotics and found it was very deficient in protein, which turns you into an airhead. The people in it were elitist and really thought they had it and were far superior.

Raw foodists believe that cooking causes food to lose most of its nutritional value; consequently, they prefer to eat uncooked foods as often as possible. Not surprisingly, many feel that vegetarians who do a good deal of cooking are missing the point in terms of health. As one said:

> I have seen and met a few regular vegetarians who looked and seemed ill. I imagine they are not getting proper nu-

> trients because they cook a lot of their vegetables. I would consign all cookbooks to the dustbin. Cooked food is dead food.

However, an ex-raw foodist had this to say about about diets based entirely on uncooked food:

> Cooking food is OK because the heat kills the toxins such as enzymes and alkaloids. Eating things like sprouts is harmful. They cause indigestion. It's best to cook sprouts. The live food theory is wrong.

The above quotations just go to show that there is no single vegetarian diet that everyone will agree upon. However, the reader should keep in mind, as we pointed out earlier, that any vegetarian diet, provided that it includes a wide variety of foods every day, is likely to be nutritionally well-balanced.

Mutual criticism also occurs among ethical vegetarians. For example, some ethical vegans are critical of animal rights supporters who are lacto-ovo-vegetarians. These people argue that lacto-ovo-vegetarians continue to include eggs and dairy products in their diets; yet, from an ethical point of view, the egg industry and the veal industry—which is a by-product of the milk industry—are among the most offensive. Ethical vegans argue that to be ethically consistent, eliminating meat is not enough; one must also stop eating dairy products and eggs.

> One thing I am surprised about is that many ethical vegetarians I have talked to will order and eat eggs in restaurants. That really bothers me because I think the poultry industry is one of the worst. I have a hard time dealing with that and I point out to them that I am surprised they're eating eggs.

In contrast, some animal rights vegetarians are critical of those who condemn nonvegetarians or nonvegans in the movement.

> So many people I know in the movement wear their vegetarianism and veganism like a badge—a status symbol. Why must they judge someone as less of an activist because they have cheese on their pizza? Not everyone may become what they are. I talk with many people and they imme-

> diately apologize about their eating habits. While I do not in any way condone the eating of animal flesh, I do not feel that I can judge them.

Finally, and somewhat surprisingly, a few vegetarians are critical of other vegetarians in general. These people feel that vegetarians, as a group, are too extreme or push their ideas too far.

> I am not joining the recipe-swapping vegetarians. Their festivities and cults do not attract me. And my wife resents the fact that she has to listen to all those eager vegetarian apostles who make a religion out of it.

> I'm a bit skeptical about some vegetarians. They have really strong ideas about various diets. And they can be very snobby. I call them "food fascists" because they are so one-way about it.

These quotations indicate some sources of tension between different types of vegetarians. Their disagreements remind us that vegetarians are not all alike; instead, they are a heterogeneous group of people with a variety of beliefs, values, and behaviors. Nevertheless, in spite of these differences, conflict is the exception rather than the rule. The great majority of vegetarians feel that regardless of a person's reasons for abstaining from meat, the implications for self, the environment, and animals are positive and worthwhile. An animal rights supporter and a health vegetarian put it this way:

> If vegetarians have reasons different from my own, that's fine. The less people are demanding meat as their major food source, the more chance we have to put a dent in factory farming and to feed all the hungry mouths on this planet. In fact, if health reasons seem to persuade people best, then health reasons should be emphasized most.

> Ethical vegetarians might not be into it for health reasons, but if they eat less animal fats and eat more fresh fruits and vegetables and whole grain products, they are bound to get healthier.

This diversity in views is not something that should be regretted. Indeed, the present popularity of a fleshless diet can largely be attributed to the fact that it appeals to a wide variety of people for diverse reasons.

SUMMARY

Earlier, we described a variety of influences that converged in the 1960s and 1970s: the health movement, a concern with spiritual values, the environmental movement, the animal rights movement, the emphasis on personal growth, and the peace movement. The accounts of individuals in this chapter reflect the impact of these social forces on people's private lives. But the melding of these various influences has meant that contemporary vegetarians are different from those of earlier eras. Vegetarians today are less likely than in the past to be motivated by narrow belief systems. Instead, they are now aware of the broad evidence that a fleshless diet is good for personal health, good for the environment, and good for the animals. In short, they have discovered that vegetarianism is a sensible and practical lifestyle well suited for the late 20th century. Modern vegetarianism is no longer a countercultural phenomenon, but an accepted variation within the mainstream of American life.

Chapter 3

The Transition to Vegetarianism

The transition to vegetarianism—during which old food habits and tastes are replaced by new vegetarian ways of eating—is a critical period. For some, the change is simple and painless. But for others it constitutes a mini-crisis. In this chapter, we explore how people go about making the transition from omnivore to herbivore. Trying to describe how people "arrive" at vegetarianism, however, is like photographing a moving object, for many people continue to change their diets, attitudes, and lifestyles long after they banish meat from their kitchens. Accordingly, it is necessary to consider not only where vegetarians come from, but where they are headed.

INITIAL INFLUENCES

Long-term vegetarians think it is normal to be vegetarian. Helen, a clinical psychologist and vegetarian for nine years, commented, "It is hard for me to remember that people still eat meat. I'm shocked when I go out with people and they order and eat it." However, most of the people we spoke with were once die-hard meat-eaters who could think of nothing better than sinking their teeth into a blood-red steak. What happened to change their minds in such a radical manner?

Exposure to the idea of vegetarianism comes about in many ways. For our respondents, these early influences fall into five broad categories. Forty percent mention other people as having had the major impact on their decisions. This is followed by books and other print media (39%), specific experiences (24%), organizational involvement (17%), and films (9%). (These percentages add to more than 100 because some people mentioned more than one influence.)

People

Vegetarians mention a variety of people who influenced their decisions to stop eating flesh. The largest group consists of friends (mentioned by 17% of all vegetarians), followed by casual acquaintances (7%); parents (4%); spouses (3%); children (3%); teachers, doctors, or other professionals (3%); extended family (2%); and siblings (1%). How do these people get the message across? In most cases, vegetarian friends and family members actively, but gently, encourage the change. This encouragement usually consists of a basic exposure to the idea, along with discussion, as the following quotations illustrate:

> I did it gradually because my Dad was health conscious and he would go to health food places. We didn't care for it that much, but once in a while we would go with him. It went gradually from there.

> I grew up in an orphanage with 50 children. One of our nurses was a vegetarian and she used to take me to her room and make little salads and talk to me about how cruel it is to kill animals. She convinced me and I have been a vegetarian since I was 11, 52 years ago.

> I was talking with a friend who was a vegan. I told him that I was more concerned with human problems than animal problems. He asked, "Would you rather eat a New Yorker you don't know or Birdie [my dog]?" I had absolutely no answer for this.

In contrast to this gentle exposure, a few people experience strong pressure from highly committed friends or family members. This pressure is often resented at the time, but it can lead to the intended outcome in the long run. For example, Lori, a counsellor, told us that her brother had a strong impact on her recent decision to stop eating meat:

> I believe I first started to think about animal issues when my brother became a Greenpeace activist and chained himself to a sealing ship in Canada and was arrested. I admired his conviction, but I had always resented his silent tension and disapproval as the rest of the family tried to enjoy a turkey dinner.

Some individuals stop eating meat after people they are living with—either roommates or family members—become vegetarian. In some cases, people willingly follow suit because they are impressed by the example set by the new vegetarian in their midst. In other cases, they change simply because it is more convenient to maintain a completely meatless household. As several people pointed out, cooking two separate meals every day quickly becomes an unnecessary chore. In a few cases, people have little choice; it comes down to a decision between giving up meat or moving out. As Leslie, a university student from England, said, "I was persuaded by my roommate to become a vegetarian. If I hadn't, she would have kicked me out of the house."

Occasionally, the first person in a household to change is a child rather than an adult. When children decide to become vegetarians, parents generally do everything they can to force them to eat meat again. Usually, parental pressure wins out and the vegetarian experiment is short-lived. But there are exceptions. The following story from Janet, a homemaker, illustrates how a shift in family eating habits was initiated by her eight-year-old daughter:

> One day we were eating a Sunday lunch—lamb—when my daughter suddenly asked, "What was this meat before you cooked it?" I told her lamb, and she announced that she wouldn't eat it because she liked lambs. She was eight and a half years old. I thought it was time to discuss vegetarianism with her. I tried to give her a balanced view but she said she no longer would eat meat. When I started cooking stuff for my daughter, I also started to eat a share of it. A year later, I decided I didn't like the idea of killing animals. So I joined my daughter in vegetarianism.

Another frequently occurring situation is for people to have their first exposure to vegetarianism while traveling with or visiting vegetarian friends or family members. After trying it for a while, these people discover they enjoy meatless cuisine, and the change becomes permanent. Steve, a business consultant, had his first exposure to meatless meals when his cousin came to visit and did a good deal of vegetarian cooking. As he said, "I thought it was silly at first, but it sparked my awareness."

Although friends and family are common influences, new acquaintances can also serve as catalysts. Some people find their curiosity is aroused after a chance encounter with a vegetarian. For example, Lona, a retired teacher, and her daughter were on a backpacking trip in Yosemite National Park when they met a young vegetarian couple. A conversation on the merits of a meatless diet started them thinking, and later they decided to decrease their own meat consumption. That was 10 years ago; today Lona, aged 70, is a semivegetarian.

A transitory meeting with a vegetarian seems unlikely to change something as fundamental as someone's diet. But this is precisely what happens to many people. How is such influence possible? In many cases, meeting a vegetarian for the first time shatters a central belief: that it is necessary to eat meat in order to live. Correspondingly, it triggers the insight that it is possible to survive in good health and in good spirits on a plant-centered diet. The following story illustrates the narrow conceptions many people hold about food and diet. Jeff, a lacto-ovo-vegetarian for 15 years, first came to reevaluate his own beliefs after meeting a member of a society where vegetarianism is common:

> I met a man from Sri Lanka who had never eaten meat in his life, nor had hardly anyone on his island, as it just wasn't part of their culture. This made me realize that a core assumption with which I had been programed all along—that one has to eat animals to live, and if you don't you wither away and die—was obviously false, as this person had lived all his life without ever taking a bite out of an animal. I think the firsthand proof pushed me into making my first move towards a flesh-free diet.

On other occasions, people are impressed by the health and attractiveness of vegetarians they meet. Some people react favorably when they are introduced to young vegetarians who are fit, muscular, and athletic. Others are surprised to meet elderly vegetarians who have the appearance and behavior of people many years younger. Julie, a beautician, had been told that a vegetarian diet might improve her hypoglycemia, but she had serious doubts about the possibility of remaining healthy without eating meat. However, she was later convinced of the soundness of a fleshless diet after an encounter with an elderly vegetarian.

> I met this 83-year-old woman who was vegetarian. I had never been exposed to it, and I thought it was crazy. But when I met this woman I was totally impressed—she had a lot of energy and vitality. She still had three businesses that she was running. Plus she had a lot of young male friends knocking on her door wanting to be in her company because of her vitality.

Sometimes the influence of other people operates in unexpected ways. For example, Elizabeth, an Australian primary school teacher, was persuaded to become vegetarian by, of all people, her butcher:

> I used to buy $150 sides of beef, whole lambs cut up, and lots of dog bones. Then the delivery man told me of seeing cows being killed and how some died slowly and how it almost made him not want to be a butcher. It put me off buying sides of beef. The occasional tuft of lamb's wool on the meat made me feel sad, but I had been brought up in a minister's family where we were taught that all meat is OK to eat. However, I now had doubts because of the butcher, and I stopped eating meat.

All in all, our research shows that vegetarianism often grows through a process of personal influence, passing from friend to friend, from family member to family member, and from acquaintance to acquaintance. This influence can take the form of direct persuasion, but it more often takes the form of information, mild encouragement, and the provision of an attractive role model. The fact that many people are influenced in such subtle ways indicates that one can bring about a good deal of change in the behavior of others simply by living as a vegetarian. Many vegetarians are probably having more influence on the people around them than they realize.

Books and Other Literature

Many people claim that printed matter was instrumental in their decisions to become vegetarian. Books are mentioned most often (by 25% of all respondents), followed by newsletters (7%), magazine or newspaper articles (4%), animal rights leaflets (2%), and academic journals (1%). Of those who mention books, three fourths refer to animal rights and animal welfare literature, and one half mention Peter Singer's work, *Animal Liberation*—the single most commonly mentioned book we encountered.

Gwen, who is active in the animal liberation movement in Australia, was strongly influenced by Singer's book. Her story reflects the fact that reading about the treatment of animals can be unpleasant, and for this reason, is often avoided. The emotional impact of this material, however, is undoubtedly a strong motivator of behavior change:

> I'd happened upon an illustrated review of Professor Peter Singer's book, *Animal Liberation*. I read the review, rushed out and bought the book, and promptly put it to rest in the book case. It was too difficult and distressing to confront. One day, a year later, I pulled up behind a truckload of pigs, obviously abattoir-bound. That clinched it. I knew that they, or others like them, would be on my plate that night. Back home, I pounced on Singer's book, read every word, and knew that I had become vegetarian.

Some ethical vegetarians also mention Tom Regan's book, *The Case for Animal Rights*, as having been influential. Because Regan's work is more academic in tone than Singer's, it tends to be of particular interest to those who have had some exposure to university level philosophy courses. Sarah received more than a good grade in her university course after becoming familiar with Regan's book:

> In 1986 I took a philosophy class that really got me started. For my class paper I decided to write on "Man's Treatment of Animals." I was having trouble finding information on the subject. Sooner or later I came across Tom Regan's book, *The Case for Animal Rights*. My term paper was a success (all 26 pages of it). Before I received my grade I had given up all meat and poultry but not fish. I soon read other books on vegetarianism, and I knew I was a lacto-vegetarian for life.

Newsletters and magazines can also be effective in changing people's behavior. For example, one issue of the *People for the Ethical Treatment of Animals News* had an immediate and powerful impact on several people we spoke with. Sherri described her reaction:

> I stopped eating meat and fish exactly one year ago, on the day I received volume one, number eight, of the publication, *PETA News*. One of the articles was titled "Downed Cow." That particular article changed my life. That entire issue was shocking, sad, and the reason I will never eat meat again.

The above quotations indicate that books and other publications are important motivators of change for some people. In addition, many people rely heavily on books and other literature for information and encouragement *after* becoming vegetarian. Books containing information on vegetarian nutrition, for example, are often sought out, as we discuss later. And new cookbooks are a necessity, as most neophytes quickly discover that their old meat-centered cookbooks are limited. Not only do traditional cookbooks have few recipes that feature plant foods as main courses, but the vegetable dishes they do include are generally unimaginative and dull. Many people report that exploring new recipes in vegetarian cookbooks is one of the most enjoyable aspects of this period.

Vegetarian literature is particularly important for those who do not know other vegetarians personally. For these people, having a subscription to a magazine such as *Vegetarian Times* or a vegetarian newsletter reduces feelings of isolation. A subscription also provides support and helps them to stick with a difficult decision when the going gets rough. Vegetarian literature not only is a catalyst for behavior change, but also plays a role in maintaining that change over time.

Specific Experiences

An anthropologist once told us a story about an experience she had had while living in an island society. The traditional diet on this island consisted of plant foods and fish, but in recent years frozen mutton had been imported from Australia. One day a group of children asked her what this meat was, assuming it must have been some sort of fish. When she explained that it was an animal and showed them a picture of a sheep, the children were horrified. To them, the thought of eating an animal that had fur was disgusting.

Many vegetarians would agree with the children in this story. And even meat-eaters often admit to feeling a bit squeamish when reminded that they regularly eat the bodies of dead animals. But most of the time, people do a good job of "forgetting" where meat comes from.

Sometimes, however, individuals have experiences that force this knowledge out of the backs of their minds and into their full awareness. As a result, they are led to reexamine their eating habits, and eventually, to give up meat. The particular experiences that produce this outcome are diverse. In our sample, the types of experiences, and the percentage of people reporting them, are: a direct insight into the nature of meat (10%), seeing food animals being transported (4%), witnessing animals being killed (3%), practicing meditation or yoga (4%), dissecting animals in a classroom (2%), and having a major illness (1%).

Insight into the Nature of Meat

A feeling of revulsion, brought on by a sudden insight into what meat is and where it comes from, is the most commonly mentioned experience. Typically, this occurs when people are eating or are about to eat. Judging from people's accounts, these "meat insight" experiences have an immediate impact on behavior.

> I stopped eating meat seven years ago abruptly when I took a bite out of a piece of barbecued chicken and found a vein sticking out, half eaten.

> A few days before I became vegetarian, I came home from school and there was a leftover roast in a pan. I saw the bone—it was a hip. And I began to think, "What am I doing? I'm eating a corpse." The whole thing became repulsive to me and I developed a dislike for meat right then.

> I had been eating tongue when I saw a cow in my mind's eye. The cow was whole. I couldn't finish the food. I quit eating all flesh.

Meat insight experiences are extremely powerful, and people often describe them in strong terms. As one person said, "It was as if a great light came on in my mind and I could suddenly see flesh-eating for what it really is: barbaric, horrible, and disgusting." These moments of insight can lead to a complete reevaluation of one's eating habits; many people become "aesthetic" vegetarians shortly afterward. As Carene put it, "The moment I realized that I was eating the furry creatures I loved, I refused to eat meat again."

In a few cases, people are confronted with the reality of flesh-eating when someone makes a joke at mealtime about meat being a dead animal. The realization that it isn't really a joke means that for the soon-to-be vegetarian, eating meat is no laughing matter.

> I was 12 when I stopped eating meat. I didn't like it. My friend stuck a fork into a leg of lamb and said "Baaa, Baaa." I quit eating all flesh after that.

> At an evening meal of homemade soup my sister joked to me, "There's a dead cow in your soup." I looked at the beef and decided that I didn't want to eat dead cows.

> I came home after class and one of my roommates said, "There's some meat in the refrigerator if you want to make

> a sandwich." I looked inside and there on a plate was a sheep fetus—my roommate's biology project. It seemed funny at the time in a macabre sort of way, but I thought about that fetus the next few times I ate meat.

Meat insight experiences can also occur when preparing or cooking meat. On these occasions, the sight, smell, or feel of raw meat causes people to associate it with a formerly living animal. An odd juxtaposition of events provided Diane, a homemaker, with an insight into what she was about to eat. Although it ruined her Thanksgiving dinner, the outcome, as far as she was concerned, was for the best:

> My husband and I were always animal lovers but for many years did not make the connection between what was on our platter and what was in our hearts. One Thanksgiving, I had to wash a turkey in the bathtub because of its size. The realization that its body was just like [that of] my dog that I washed in the same tub was overwhelming. We became vegetarians that night.

Food insight experiences sometimes have unusual origins. One woman told us about a nightmare she had had about eating meat. The day before, she had bought some meat from a butcher shop, and the sound of hacking while she was standing in line made an impression on her. That night, she had a nightmare about a cow being sliced up and served while still alive. The next day she became a vegetarian. In her case, she had been uncomfortable with the idea of eating animals for some time; the nightmare was simply a reflection of her growing anxiety over eating flesh.

Another unusual story comes from a mother who became a vegetarian after having to explain the origin of meat to her young daughter. Being forced to confront the truth led her to perceive the chicken on her plate, not as her dinner, but as a dead animal:

> My family was sitting down to a meal of fried chicken and my young daughter brought her toy chicken to the table with her. My husband's aunt said, "Eat your chicken." My daughter seemed surprised at these words. She looked at

her aunt, her toy chicken, and then at her plate. At that moment I realized that I would have to explain to my child where meat comes from. How could I tell this innocent child who loved animals so dearly that her own mother and father actually fed on slaughtered cows, pigs, and chickens? All at once the sight of the dead chicken on my plate nauseated me. I realized that I was deeply ashamed of the fact that I ate meat. I knew the only answer was for me to become vegetarian and to raise my daughter as one as well.

Some of the saddest stories we heard were from people who, as children, had their pets dished up for dinner. As one person said, "I first seriously decided to do without meat when my mother cooked my pet rabbit in a stew and I ate it without knowing it." Another person came home from school one day, looked in the refrigerator, and saw a rabbit sliced up on a plate. She asked her mother, "Is this my rabbit?" It was. Surely, nothing can drive home more clearly to children the connection between the meat on their plates and a living animal than to see their own pets cooked and served.

It is curious that meat insight experiences are not more common than they are. Many people, for example, handle meat every day when cooking; yet, the sight and smell of blood do not repulse them. Perhaps individuals who are disgusted by meat simply have "weak" stomachs. However, this seems unlikely. Many people who touch meat (which is muscle tissue and fat) without qualms would feel queasy about manipulating the intestines, brains, or eyes of the same animal. And handling the flesh of a dog or cat would probably disgust many people in the United States, even though these animals are considered food sources in other parts of the world. Even internal organs considered to be food in our culture, such as beef tongue, tripe, oxtail, and brains, are eaten only by a minority of people.

These observations reflect the fact that humans "compartmentalize" their thinking. This allows animals defined as food and those not defined as food to be perceived differently. Psychologists are aware that people use a variety of defenses and rationalizations to protect themselves from the unpleasant implications of their behavior. In the case of meat-eating, people use *denial* to convince themselves that beef, veal, pork, chicken, and lamb are not really the bodies of animals. People also have an almost magical belief that cooking transforms raw flesh from something that is completely unpalatable into something that is edible—as if the application of heat transforms the body of an animal into a steak, a hamburger, or a drumstick. In spite of the current penchant for sushi, most people would cringe at the prospect of eating a raw pot roast.

These tendencies are reinforced by advertising and the meat industry. For example, old-fashioned butcher shops once posted pictures of steers with dotted lines superimposed on their bodies delineating the various cuts of meat, with images of roasts, steaks, and ribs decorating the borders. However, marketing studies revealed that these charts were offensive to many shoppers; people didn't want to be reminded that they were eating animals. Consequently, these images are rarely seen in the meat sections of modern supermarkets.

Witnessing the Killing of Animals

Similar to meat insight experiences are occasions on which people witness the slaughtering of animals. Some individuals are so upset after seeing animals being killed that they stop eating meat on the spot. In some cases, this experience occurs during childhood. For example, the following woman, now 35, became vegetarian when she was five years old:

> I was visiting my grandparents on the farm. I remember being real upset by it. I saw the whole process from the animal being alive and petting it [to] then seeing it butchered. I have vague memories of it now, but I remember it happening and refusing to have anything to do with eating animals after that.

People who are raised on farms have a good deal of exposure to farm animals. Having the opportunity to experience an emotional bond with an animal, only to see it later sent to slaughter, can result in a strong predisposition to vegetarianism later in life. Jenny, a dietician, recounted a particularly painful experience from her past:

> I was raised on a farm and did not like killing chickens from an early age. I exhibited a champion Black Angus 4-H calf who cried when I left it. Actually, we both cried. I knew then that he knew what was in store for him. I didn't eat meat for a long time after that.

The above accounts suggest that children are especially sensitive to the killing of animals. Perhaps this is because they, unlike adults, have not yet been strongly conditioned into believing that slaughtering and eating animals is normal and appropriate. Over time, the ability of most children to empathize with animals becomes blunted by a culture that treats animals largely as objects to be used.

For many adults, however, the sight of animals being slaughtered can be just as upsetting as it is for children. A visit to a slaughterhouse, in particular, is a grim experience that can make a vegetarian out of the hardiest meat-eater. The following woman visited a slaughterhouse to find out for herself what happens:

> I decided to take a visit to one of the abattoirs just down the road from where I lived at the time. The smell of blood and fear made me so ill I had to cut my visit short. [I] went out to the car and threw up, and cried for ages. I have not eaten meat since that day.

If the impact of slaughterhouses is so powerful, then how do people manage to work in them and continue to eat meat? First, there is probably self-selection occurring, such that workers who are sensitive to the suffering of animals quit after a short time and find employment elsewhere. Secondly, after working in a slaughterhouse for a period of time, most people become emotionally desensitized. Although the first few hours and days might be difficult, after witnessing thousands of animals being killed, even a sympathetic person would exhibit little emotional reaction. Nevertheless, we encountered a couple of ex-slaughterhouse workers who later became vegetarians, so not everyone is able to habituate to the daily carnage.

Given the emotional impact of visiting a slaughterhouse, it seems likely that many people would become vegetarian if animals were killed and processed in supermarket parking lots instead of behind closed doors in remote country areas. For some people, however, witnessing the slaughter of animals is not necessary; merely the sight of animals being transported to slaughter—a common experience in rural areas—is the final straw. One respondent, an English Rastafarian, had already taken the first tentative steps toward giving up meat when he had an unsettling experience. As he said, "During a car ride following a cattle truck, a cow looked straight into my eyes, and I was certain it knew that it was going to its death." After that, he became a vegetarian.

Two individuals in our sample were influenced by the killing of companion animals. One man, a university student, worked for a time as a veterinarian's assistant and had the unpleasant duty of euthanizing animals. Similarly, a woman who managed an animal shelter became concerned about the "massive killing of healthy pets and ex-pets." For her, vegetarianism "helps to compensate for all the animals I must kill as part of my job."

Classroom Biology Dissections

Some people have experiences in high school or college classrooms that lead them to consider vegetarianism. Although biology class dissections often desensitize students to the needs of animals or to their ability to experience pain, the opposite also occurs, as in the following story:

> I became a vegetarian when I was a sophomore in high school. I was motivated to do so by a biology class project where I had to dissect a fetal pig. The pigs that the class dissected had been taken from their mothers' wombs when their mothers had been slaughtered. This project made me realize the cruelty of killing animals for food.

Having an Operation

Perhaps the most unexpected experience was that of two people who became vegetarians after experiencing an illness. For these people, experiencing pain, and contemplating their own mortality, led to a new sympathy for the plight of animals. Belinda told us that after an operation for cervical cancer, she came to realize "how precious all life is." Lester, an English vegan, told us his story:

> Four years ago I went into hospital for an operation on polyps in my bladder. I went through terrible, agonizing spasms of pain. I came out of hospital and for a year or more thought about that terrible pain. I got to thinking about animals. I got to realizing that millions of animals were suffering that same terrible pain that I had felt. So I went vegetarian.

Meditation and Yoga

The experiences that impel most people to give up meat-eating are unpleasant. In contrast, meditation and yoga provide attractive and enjoyable routes to vegetarianism for a few people. Practitioners of these disciplines often say that a meatless diet is a natural and inevitable step; many claim that the adoption of a vegetarian diet under these circumstances is effortless and "just seems to happen."

> I was taking a yoga class and it felt perfect to me. I eagerly practiced the exercises on my own as well as in class. Slowly the desire to eat meat and put harmful substances into my body vanished. It was easy.

Why should people doing meditation and yoga lose their desire to eat flesh? Most likely, this is due to the fact that these practices require people to spend a good deal of time attending closely to their bodies. With their attention focused on how they are feeling, they realize that a meal based on flesh and animal fat often leaves them feeling sluggish. This is because animal products take a longer time to digest than do fruits, vegetables, and other plant foods. And to the extent that well-balanced vegetarian meals lead to improvements in energy and mood (as we discuss later), the desire to enhance one's well-being through a good diet should be reinforced.

Organizations

Some people become vegetarians through their involvement in groups or organizations that require or recommend vegetarianism. The two major types of organizations represented in our sample are animal rights organizations (mentioned by 10% of all respondents) and religious groups (mentioned by 7% of respondents). Religious groups with vegetarian elements include the Seventh-Day Adventists, the International Society for Krishna Consciousness, and followers of Sri Chinmoy or other Eastern religious teachers. In most cases, people are attracted to the group for religious reasons and adopt vegetarianism shortly after joining.

In recent years, animal welfare organizations have been directing more of their attention to issues involving farm animals. This change in emphasis has led many to encourage their members to practice vegetarianism. Consequently, many individuals give up meat shortly after joining one of these groups. However, for some people, particularly those who have been involved in animal welfare activities for a long time, the relation between compassion for animals and vegetarianism takes many years to "sink in." These contrasting lengths of time are illustrated in the following two quotations:

> I became involved in the animal welfare movement and immediately saw a conflict between saving cats and killing cows. I read a flyer that stated if I ate chicken twice a week, I was guilty of killing that chicken. At that instant, my consciousness changed and I knew that I was not capable of harming or killing an animal just for its flesh and couldn't justify having someone else do it for me.
>
> I had been actively and profoundly involved in animal welfare work for approximately twenty years. It suddenly oc-

> curred to me one day that my eating habits and my animal-related activities were incongruous. I began to question how I would fight so hard to protect animals with one hand and stick a knife and fork in them with the other.

As the above quotation suggests, a belief in animal welfare alone is often insufficient to get people to stop eating meat. For many, a little extra motivation is necessary. Some animal rights supporters experience pressure from others in the movement to become vegetarian. This pressure—sometimes subtle and sometimes strong and direct—leads many to bring their eating habits in line with their ideologies.

Occasionally, however, pressure from people outside the movement does the trick. A typical situation is one in which, during an argument over animal rights, animal advocates are confronted with the inconsistency between their beliefs and their meat-eating behavior. The realization that their opponents are correct is a strong incentive for these people to take the first step toward vegetarianism. Joan, for example, had a disagreement with her boss, a doctor, about the use of animals in medical experiments. During their discussion, he pointed out the conflict between her professed interest in animal rights and her diet. His comments led her to realize that she was indeed acting inconsistently in treating food animals differently from other animals. Today Joan is an ethical vegan. As she said, "I'm glad he pointed it out to me."

Films

Sometimes a film or video is responsible for a change to vegetarianism. Occasionally, the influence of films is very indirect. For example, after watching the "Kung Fu" TV series, Ray became interested in Zen Buddhism, and through that, vegetarianism. In most cases, however, the impact of a film is immediate, particularly if the film depicts animal suffering or slaughter. Some people, for example, become upset after watching films about the food or fur industries on television. These films, it seems, can be educational on a moral as well as a factual level.

> I saw a special on PBS on slaughterhouses and it really affected me. They showed one of the cows going to slaughter and it had tears in its eyes. I made a declaration at that point that I was going to be vegetarian.
>
> When I was 13 years old I saw a program on TV on the harp seal slaughter. I shall never forget seeing the seal pup as it was clubbed to death, and the way the mother followed the hunters as they dragged the carcass along the ice. I have never eaten, nor used, animal products since.

Other people are strongly influenced by films with a specific vegetarian message, such as *Vegetarian World,* narrated by William Shatner, and *The Animals Film* (a film about the treatment of animals by the meat, cosmetics, and medical research industries). Some people mention watching videos on vegetarianism after enjoying a meatless meal at Govindas restaurants, which are run by the International Society for Krishna Consciousness.

Although mentioned less often than other sources, films can have a powerful impact when viewed under the right circumstances. The power of film derives from the sense of immediacy and reality conveyed by the visual image. Clearly, it is one thing to read about animal suffering, and something else to see it. The following story from Janice, vegetarian and freelance writer, illustrates the power of visual images to change opinions:

> Hearing that *The Animals Film,* a documentary depicting various ways in which humans abuse and exploit nonhumans, including graphic footage of factory farming and animals being slaughtered, was going to be aired on our local public station, I told my parents of it and asked them if they would please try to watch it, knowing that they probably couldn't handle watching the whole thing, but hoping that they might watch even a bit of it. They did watch all of it, to my surprise. My mother told me that it upset my father greatly for many days afterward. He is in his sixties, as is my mother; both have eaten meat all their lives. My previous efforts to talk to them about vegetarianism, and to be an example of a happy, healthy, well-adjusted person who chooses not to eat meat, had been met with indifference

> and even some skepticism on my father's part. But, to make a long story shorter, my mother next informed me after we had been to the supermarket that my father had decreed that he would have no more meat in his house, nor would he eat any anywhere else. So, this wonderful film helped to make two new ethical vegetarians! It was one of the happiest days of my life.

MAKING THE CHANGE

The time taken to make the transition from being a meat-eater to a vegetarian varies considerably. Some stop immediately on the day they decide to become vegetarians while others eliminate meat from their diets over periods of months or even years. A gradual phasing out of meat is the most common approach, with 70 percent of people taking this route and 30 percent giving up meat all at once.

The Quick Change

Individuals who give up meat suddenly fall into four categories. First, those who have experiences that evoke strong emotional reactions change quickly. Meat insight experiences, for example, can produce feelings of disgust that lead people to become vegetarians on the spot. Others feel such moral outrage after learning about conditions on factory farms that they vow without further consideration never to eat meat again. Mike, a high school English teacher, told us that he had never considered vegetarianism before receiving an issue of *PETA News* dealing with farm animals:

> I quit on the spot, totally. Before I received that issue (out of the blue I might add—I must have been on a mailing list) I had eaten a cheeseburger for lunch. When I got up from my reading chair I was a vegetarian and haven't eaten another creature's body since.

Second, some people want to become vegetarian for a period of time but confront practical barriers that make it difficult for them to stop eating meat. In these cases, people turn vegetarian as soon as their circumstances change. Typical situations are ones in which young adults are living with meat-eating parents or in dormitories. In other cases, people become vegetarians after separating from meat-eating spouses.

Third, some individuals plan on becoming vegetarians for a period of time, but wait for a day that implies a clear demarcation between one period and the next to begin. Some people begin their vegetarian diets as a New Year's Eve resolution. Two of our respondents chose Meat Boycott Week to make the change. And moving was a good cutting point for Robyn:

> The decision to make a commitment to vegetarianism as part of a more general commitment to animals came upon me suddenly. I was moving from one apartment to another, and my brother was helping me. Since our kitchen things were packed up, he went out and got some fast-food fried chicken. I ate the greasy stuff and then announced, "That's it. No more." The repugnance I felt was both physical and moral.

Fourth, a few people think about vegetarianism for a long time, but do little about it. Then, on a day when they finally feel ready, they announce to the world, and to themselves, that they are vegetarians. For these people, the time simply has to be right. As Janine put it, "Since childhood, I was always bothered by the thought of eating animals. One day, out of nowhere, I decided that I had a choice. I stopped completely."

The Gradual Change

As noted earlier, most people make the transition to vegetarianism by gradually eliminating flesh foods from their diets. These periods of time range, in our sample, from one month to four years, with one year being the median amount of time taken. There is a typical pattern to this transition, with 79 percent giving up red meat first, followed by chicken and fish at a later point in time. Some of these people give up red meat and chicken quickly, but continue to eat fish for a relatively long period of time. Another 12 percent gradually cut down on all types of meat simultaneously. (In addition, one person who developed an aversion to meat while gnawing on chicken legs gave those up first, one person concerned about the clubbing of baby seals gave up fish first, and one person gave up veal first.)

Quite a few people are eating less meat these days than they did in the past. Consequently, some individuals notice that their diets have been gradually evolving in the direction of vegetarianism for a long period of time. When these people finally decide to become full vegetarians, the transition is relatively easy because they are already halfway toward their goal. The experience of Martha, a homemaker and mother, illustrates this pattern:

> I wanted to get my family off the "ground beef merry-go-round" for health reasons. I had stopped cooking beef and I never bought pork. I made recipes using small portions of chicken and other low fat products. I was trying to get the fat out of our diet. Looking back, I realize that I was heading in the direction of vegetarianism all along. I had taken several steps already, so the final one to a nonflesh lifestyle was easy.

One might predict that people with a strong ethical basis for their beliefs would be more likely to make a quick transition than would those who reject meat for reasons of health or personal growth. However, there does not appear to be any relation between people's motives for being vegetarian and the length of time it takes them to change. Ethical vegetarians, in fact, often take a relatively long period of time to completely purge flesh from their diets. It seems surprising that the following person took so long to change, considering the strength of her convictions. But her story is not atypical.

> For the past two years, I had been heavily involved in the Animal Rights Movement. In April, 1984, I was one of the first fifteen people ever arrested in the United States during an act of civil disobediance on behalf of animals. I had been arrested, brought to trial, and convicted. I had been in dem-

onstrations, on the picket line, and had written letters until worn out. But it took me a full two years before I stopped eating dead animals. I wonder sometimes why it took me a while, particularly since I knew the truth about where the flesh came from.

THE BENEFITS OF BEING PREPARED

Is it hard to stop eating meat? For most people, the answer is "No." About three fourths of our respondents (73%) claim that the transition is not difficult, although many experience some degree of inconvenience or awkwardness. The ease with which the transition is made partly depends on how well prepared people are. Among people who had prepared themselves by reading and trying out recipes, 80 percent describe the transition as easy. But among those who were not prepared, only 56 percent describe the transition as easy.

The majority of people (61%) become vegetarian before they know anything about vegetarian cooking, and most are unfamiliar with the wide range of nontraditional foods that make vegetarian cuisine so diverse and interesting. Many continue to cook as they used to, boiling vegetables until they turn into mush and serving them with a potato. Some branch out and try brown rice, but don't realize that it takes a little longer to cook than white rice does. No doubt, many of the first nonmeat meals prepared by novice vegetarians are appalling. Concoctions of soggy vegetables and undercooked brown rice or beans are enough to critically test the morale and willpower of even the most committed vegetarian.

> I wasn't well prepared. There was a lack of recipes and a lack of awareness of how to cook differently. All of a sudden I was left without anything to stick in the skillet.

> I wasn't prepared. I didn't know what to eat. It was strange. I remember cabbage soup—it was so bland. I thought, "If this is what it is like, I don't know if I can do this."

Many people wander through natural food stores or health food shops in search of vegetarian products they have heard about, such as tofu, tempeh, or miso. Others look closely at the imported and specialty foods available in conventional supermarkets. However, for people raised on meat-and-potatoes diets, these new vegetarian foods can be confusing. Many people don't know how to cook with soy products and find their taste unappealing. Even plain and humble foods, such as lentils, seem "exotic" to some and are a complete conundrum to others. As Suzanne, a vegetarian for one year, described it:

> I was in the dark. I read a vegetarian cookbook, but the ingredients in the recipes seemed so far out. I felt truly foreign in the natural foods store. Words like legumes and tamari seemed unreal to me. We were eating pasta and pizza for quite some time.

After a period of eating mediocre food, most people set about learning how to prepare tasty vegetarian meals. This often requires a change in ideas about food. Most people grow up with the idea that everything other than meat falls into the category of "side dish." But after a while, people begin to see that a grain (such as rice pilaf) or a particular vegetable (such as stuffed pumpkin) can serve as the basis of a satisfying main course. Considering that there are only a few types of meats, but dozens of different types of vegetables, grains, legumes, nuts, and seeds, it is clear that vegetarian cuisine is anything but limited. Eventually, new vegetarians outgrow the feeling that a meal without meat is incomplete. As Joan said:

> I didn't know anything. All I did was cook the same stuff and leave the meat out. It wasn't very satisfying. So it took a shift in thinking and practice to learn to cook meatless dishes. I bought some cookbooks, got a subscription to *Vegetarian Times,* and talked to my vegetarian friends. I went to their houses and saw what they ate. Then I found a brand of tofu "hot dogs" and I couldn't eat enough of them. I loved them. Once I found them my problem was essentially over.

Some individuals spend a lot of time reading about nutrition before becoming vegetarian. In some cases, people do this because the idea of a change in diet stimulates their interest in matters related to food and nutrition. In other cases, they are worried that they might damage their health by omitting meat from their diets. These people's fears spring from a lifetime of having been told that meat is necessary for good health. And many are warned by family members or friends that they will become anemic or get sick if they stop eating meat. Some believe that vegetarians have to be eternally vigilant to ensure that they get enough protein or other nutrients. For these reasons, it is not uncommon for new vegetarians to be anxious about the adequacy of their diets.

> I knew that when you change diets, you can't do it on your own; you have to know what you are doing, especially with something like vegetarianism. I was afraid that I wouldn't get the proper food balance, so I joined a nutrition class and read books. I believed that you couldn't just become vegetarian because you wanted to—you need guidance.

Although many new vegetarians are concerned about nutrition, most find that a little reading on the topic helps to put their minds at ease. Their fears are further put to rest when they seek out and meet people who have been vegetarians for 10 or 20 years and are in good health. And, for many, their own feelings of physical and psychological well-being after adopting a meatless diet are the final proof that they are on the right track. Consequently, many vegetarians feel that fears about dietary deficiencies are overexaggerated. They claim that of all people, vegetarians are the ones with the *least* need to be concerned about nutrition. As one person stated:

> I wasn't prepared at all. And I still don't think you have to be prepared. I don't think becoming vegetarian is a health hazard or that you have to be careful. Meat-eaters are the ones who should be worrying.

As we described earlier, vegetarians have little difficulty in meeting the current recommended dietary guidelines. But it is still necessary to eat sensibly. Consequently, increasing one's knowledge about nutrition is always useful, regardless of whether one is on a vegetarian or a meat-centered diet.

A number of people in our sample, because they were unprepared and didn't know what to cook, ate poorly after giving up flesh foods. For example, one person lived exclusively on junk food and peanut butter and jelly sandwiches on white bread for the first six months. Several people who lived for a period of time on poor-quality vegetarian diets claimed that they didn't feel particularly healthy, which is not surprising. Their level of health and sense of well-being improved, however, when they improved the quality of their diets.

Some individuals are largely indifferent to food—something which is difficult for those of us who love to eat to understand. For these people, giving up meat was "no big deal," and they are no more concerned about the quality of their meals or their health as vegetarians than they had been as meat-eaters. Andy, for example, was unprepared when he gave up eating meat, but felt that no preparation was necessary. As he put it:

> It was easy for me because I didn't care about food too much in general. I didn't know a damn thing about nutrition or health. I wasn't interested in the health aspects. I'm not even sure I knew there were any. Sort of a blind leap. My attitude was, "I'd rather be an unhealthy vegetarian than continue eating these animals." My favorite kinds of meat were the rankest. I stopped on a dime with a stale bologna sandwich.

Our results suggest that most people who are serious about vegetarianism adapt well over time, regardless of how well prepared they are. But being familiar with vegetarian cooking and nutrition prior to eliminating meat helps to make the transition smoother and worry-free. Of course, it is also possible to learn on the job. At one point or another most people find it useful, and fun, to read up on vegetarian cooking, nutrition, and philosophy.

JUST ONE MORE STEAK

A question commonly asked of vegetarians is, "Don't you miss eating meat?" To people whose lives consist of filling in time between one hamburger and the next, the idea of never eating meat again seems about as appealing as lifelong celibacy or solitary confinement. In fact, many vegetarians do miss the flavor and texture of meat, and many find the early weeks and months to be difficult. However, people change, and after a period of time, most wonder how they ever managed to eat the stuff in the first place.

Initial Cravings

Because most of us are raised as meat-eaters, and because our culture places a high social value on meat, it is not surprising that many new vegetarians have a continuing desire for flesh foods. About half (48%) experience cravings for meat and have difficulty with the thought of giving it up forever. Interestingly, women are as likely as men to report these cravings—a finding that contradicts the notion that men are more attached to meat than are women. Ethical vegetarians are also as likely as health vegetarians to have strong yearnings for meat, suggesting that it is easier to change one's mind than one's taste buds.

> The first year that I was vegetarian I remember that my mouth used to literally water at the sight of meat cooking or being eaten. It was hard to resist and I really had to control myself.
>
> It wasn't easy at first. There is no one in the world who loved cheeseburgers and steaks more than I did. I was raised on steaks. At a restaurant that's all I ever ordered, a T-bone or a Filet Mignon. But my convictions changed me.

Not knowing how to prepare tasty vegetarian meals exacerbates this problem; boiled cabbage and mashed potatoes are unlikely to be satisfying to a person whose mouth is watering for a beef enchilada or a pizza with pepperoni. Not surprisingly, people who are not well prepared tend to experience greater cravings for meat. But as they learn how to prepare and appreciate vegetarian foods (such as tofu enchiladas or vegetarian pizza), the cravings become less severe.

Because food is so closely associated with our social and emotional lives, the thought of some meats can evoke a sense of nostalgia for pleasant times or social occasions. Traditional Thanksgiving and Christmas dinners—complete with turkeys or hams—are closely associated with fond memories of family gatherings. The smell of frying bacon in the morning reminds some people of cozy, safe days at home as a child. And the smell of barbecues is closely linked to memories of enjoyable summer holidays. As one person put it, "The hardest thing for me to give up was barbecues. In summertime the smell of barbecues was tough for a while."

Some people experience a sense of loss, as if these times can no longer be re-created. Some even feel angry because these personally meaningful events from the past are so strongly associated with the eating of flesh. However, most vegetarians discover that it is possible to continue to enjoy these rituals by replacing the meat with vegetarian alternatives. For example, vegetarian barbecues, including soyburgers with all the trimmings, help many vegetarians to realize they have no reason to feel deprived. The same principle applies to holidays. Many vegetarians regularly stage elaborate Thanksgiving or Christmas dinners for family and friends, complete with a variety of gourmet meatless dishes.

Fast foods are missed by many people, be it the hamburger or hot dog in America, the fish and chips in England, or the meat pie in Australia. The numerous associations these foods have with social occasions (such as sharing a pizza with friends) makes them emotionally important. Many also miss the convenience of fast foods. Interestingly, one common fantasy among vegetarians is the wish to open a meatless fast-food restaurant.

Fortunately for new vegetarians, many companies are now producing reasonable vegetarian analogues to meat-based fast foods, such as tofu hot dogs and tempeh burgers. These are not only convenient and help to satisfy cravings, but also are of better nutritional quality than those based on meat (they typically have less cholesterol, fat, calories, and sodium). Many vegetarians, of course, would argue that these foods also *taste* better than the flesh foods on which they are modeled. In spite of their attractions, these foods are generally not available in fast-food restaurants, so vegetarians have to purchase them in specialty shops and take them home to prepare—a major limitation for people who need to eat on the run.

We spoke with a number of people who had embarked on vegetarian diets within the last year and were currently struggling with meat cravings. These people often describe long lists of foods they continue to long for, and many clearly feel deprived. Those who have been vegetarians for a long time, or for whom the initial transition was easy, may underestimate the amount of difficulty some people have in abstaining from flesh.

> I loved the taste of meat and fish, and I still do today. I never ate steaks and hamburgers, but to this day I greatly miss meatloaf, roast, cold cuts, bacon, sausages, ham, and especially gravies derived from them.

> I have not stopped craving meat at all. I would still enjoy it. The smell of Sunday lunch still drives me crazy. I look forward to the time when scientists can reproduce the exact flavors and texture of meat. I have found nothing to come anywhere near the delicious tang of meat in its appeal.

These feelings do not always go away, and some people continue to experience cravings for years. The following comments are from people who had been completely vegetarian for two and three years, respectively:

> I have to admit that despite it all, nothing beats the taste of meat, fish, or chicken. It will take me a long time to get over my cravings for the flavor of these foods.

> I miss fried chicken, hamburgers, and bacon. I would never have become a vegetarian for health reasons alone, unless a doctor pronounced a death sentence if I didn't.

Although occasional cravings for meat can persist for long periods of time, the satisfaction people receive from living in accordance with their principles usually more than compensates for the slight inconvenience. A vegetarian of nine years made the following comment:

> I find I still miss the taste of meat. Whenever I smell it cooking, I get a little tinge of regret. But that is shortly replaced with a feeling of relief at not supporting animal slavery and slaughter.

Although cravings for meat are common, most people (52%) report no problems with them. Some people do not miss meat because they never liked it much in the first place. But in most cases, people who enjoyed eating meat are surprised to find, contrary to their expectations, that they don't miss it at all.

> I was in love with meat and wouldn't have given it up for just health reasons. But I had no trouble adapting to the instant change. I had no physical complaints or withdrawals in giving up meat.

> There was no difficulty in giving up meat. There has never been a time when I thought that I would like a hamburger, because I would have had it if I felt like it. It has never been an issue or a deprivation.

Giving In

Occasionally, vegetarians give in to sudden cravings for meat. This is not uncommon among recent converts during the first year or two. In most cases, it involves fast food such as hamburgers, hot dogs, or pizzas—the foods most likely to be purchased and eaten impulsively.

How do people react to eating flesh again? Some people find that these foods taste good at the time, but negative physical reactions shortly follow.

> Once I succumbed to the smell of meat cooking and had a burger. It tasted good, it smelled good, but I felt terrible. I felt that this was a clear indication that my body was saying, "Nah, we're tired of this."

> Approximately one year after giving up meat, at an all day picnic, I was extremely hungry, hot, and tired. I had only

> eaten an ear of corn all day and by late afternoon, with the aid of coaxing from my friend's family that it would be all right "just this once," I broke down and ate a hot dog. I was sick afterward—emotionally and physically. I had an upset stomach, and worse, I had sold out my beliefs.

It is difficult to say whether these negative physical reactions are due to indigestion or a guilty conscience—or both. Nevertheless, these experiences typically help to strengthen the resolve and commitment of most people.

Feelings about Eating Meat Now

Although initial cravings for meat are common, they typically fade with the passing of time—usually within six months to a year. As noted above, only a handful of the vegetarians we spoke with were still experiencing cravings, and most of these were recent converts. After a period of time, even former meat-lovers come to find the sight, and particularly the smell, of meat to be nauseating. The following comments are from people who experienced strong cravings during the early days of their transition:

> Vegetarianism gets easier all the time. The farther away I get from flesh-eating, the more repulsive it seems.

> Now the smell of a hamburger cooking turns my stomach, and I do not like going into restaurants. The business of dining strikes me as somewhat decadent, especially when the dined-upon are dead animals.

> In this stage of my conversion, I can't stand the smell of any flesh food and become nauseated at the thought of eating it.

To further explore this issue, we asked people how they would feel about eating meat now. This turned out to be one of the few questions on which a clear majority emerged: Eighty-two percent of vegetarians say there is no way they would consider eating flesh again. Feelings of disgust at the very thought of eating meat are prominent in most people's responses. To many, the idea is simply unthinkable.

> Just the idea of greasiness, and knowing what meat is. I just can't even imagine eating it.
>
> I don't even think about it. It is so natural to me to be vegetarian.
>
> The thought of eating an animal's corpse is very offensive to me now.

Some people are particularly adamant about never eating meat again. For example, one person said, "You couldn't get me to eat meat with a gun to my head." Another said, "Someone could pay me a million dollars and I wouldn't do it." Typically, these people have been vegetarian for a relatively long period of time. To them, eating meat has become an impossibility.

Some people no longer think of meat as food. For example, one person said that his eating meat would be equivalent to a meat-eater eating wood; it simply is not an edible thing as far as he is concerned. Along similar lines, others feel that eating meat is a form of cannibalism; consequently, they don't think about eating animal flesh any more than the average person contemplates eating another human being. For example, Mary, a social worker, said, "If you offered me meat, I'd feel the same as if you barbecued my next door neighbor and offered me a piece of his flesh—totally repulsed." For those ethical and spiritual vegetarians who feel a deep bond with animals, the use of the term "cannibalism" is more than a metaphor—it reflects a belief that the eating of animal flesh and the eating of human flesh are equally barbaric.

In spite of the fact that most vegetarians feel so strongly about never eating meat again, a minority (17%) say they might under certain circumstances. For example, a few claim they will politely eat meat if it is served to them by relatives. And a few recent converts admit that they wouldn't mind trying some of their favorite meat dishes again. Jamie, a raw foodist, said that people shouldn't make a "religion" out of vegetarianism and that he would have no qualms about eating meat again if he had the urge. However, he pointed out that if he were to eat meat, it would have to be raw!

In summary, for most people, the transition to vegetarianism is a major life change. Initially, the novelty can be overwhelming. Many new vegetarians are not 100 percent confident that they have made the right decision and have doubts about their willpower. Some anticipate symptoms of meat withdrawal or near starvation because they don't know what to cook. Others worry that they will become weak and anemic. And most feel awkward calling themselves "vegetarians" when only a short time ago they were gnawing on drumsticks. Giving up flesh involves more than simply buying a new cookbook; it involves a major shift in one's self-concept and lifestyle. As part of this process, new vegetarians have to relearn many of their beliefs, attitudes, and behavior.

However, at the same time, there is a sense of adventure, and fun, in becoming a vegetarian. And typically, over the course of a year or so, people adapt. They learn how to cook, establish new eating habits, and lose their anxiety about whether or not they made the right choice. At a certain point, the inevitable happens: People become "real" vegetarians. After this, it feels normal to abstain from flesh, and, without any self-consciousness, people define themselves as vegetarians. When someone looks at a steak and thinks, "My God. How can people eat that stuff?," it is clear that the transition has been successful.

CHANGES IN VEGETARIANS' DIETS

A vegetarian diet is not static. People try out new foods and dishes, and in the process, drop some and retain others. People also adopt different types of diets, and may experiment with macrobiotics, fruitarianism, natural hygiene, or other styles of eating. And, of course, people move from less restrictive to more restrictive diets: from semivegetarianism to lacto-ovo-vegetarianism, from lacto-ovo-vegetarianism to veganism, and in some cases, from veganism to diets based on raw foods.

We asked people not only about their present diets, but also about any changes they wished to make. Most people, as it turns out, are happy with their diets just as they are. But about one fifth want to change. For them, the present diet is a temporary stage on the way to an ideal diet.

Those who wish to change fall into three groups. First, some semivegetarians (who eat fish occasionally) plan to become full-fledged vegetarians. These are usually people who have been modifying their diets slowly, but feel the time is ready to go one step further. As one person said, "I will have to give up fish soon. I feel guilty eating it."

Second, some lacto-ovo-vegetarians want to decrease their dependence on high-fat, high-cholesterol animal products. A common pattern is for people to increase their consumption of cheese and eggs shortly after becoming vegetarians to compensate for the loss of meat. This is done for two reasons. First, familiar dishes based on dairy products and eggs, such as macaroni and cheese, cheese enchiladas, quiches, and omelettes, help to make the transition easier for many people. Second, many people consume these foods daily because they are concerned about getting sufficient protein. But because these products contain large amounts of animal fat and cholesterol, the health advantages of a meatless diet are partly negated. Over time, however, they consume dairy products and eggs less often and learn to use soy products, beans, lentils, and other high-protein foods in main courses.

Third, some vegetarians wish to adopt a completely vegan diet. Some wish to do this for health reasons, as noted above, whereas others are motivated by moral concerns. They realize that from an ethical perspective, the egg and dairy industries present serious problems. As noted earlier, battery hens are treated harshly in modern factory farms—debeaked and crowded into small cages where they do not have room even to spread their wings. Many dairy cows spend their lives tethered in small stalls where they have minimal room to move. Even more problematic is the fact that the veal industry is a by-product of the dairy industry. Dairy cows must give birth at frequent intervals in order to provide milk, and their male offspring are generally used for veal. Knowledge of the interconnections between dairy products and the veal industry leads most ethical vegetarians to consider, at some point in time, becoming vegan. Many would like to take the next step, but see a rocky road ahead. As Colette said:

> I still eat cheese and dairy products, which I love. Although it was very easy to quit eating meat, it will be much harder to eliminate dairy products from my diet. I used to think dairy products were OK because animals were not killed to make them, but lately I have been reading articles that say that animals suffer because of the dairy industry, so I guess I will have to try to give them up too. But, as I say, it will be hard.

Finally, some lacto-vegetarians and vegans try to increase the proportion of uncooked foods in their diets. This is based on the belief that cooking foods reduces their nutritional value. Fred, the owner of a popular restaurant, was making an effort to include raw foods in every meal. As he said, "I've reached a point now where a meal doesn't seem like a meal unless it has a salad with it."

Lacto-ovo-vegetarians who hope to become vegans cite four potential problems that hold them back. First, many hold strong emotional attachments to familiar foods and dishes that require dairy products or eggs. This, of course, is the same problem that many people face in rejecting meat, as we noted earlier. Foods that people frequently mention, in addition to milk and cheese, are butter, half-and-half in coffee, cream, yogurt, ice cream, and baked goods with eggs. As the above list suggests, one of the chief attractions of dairy products is fat; many people crave the taste of fat and find it difficult to give up.

Second, some people claim they would be willing to give up dairy products and eggs if suitable substitutes were available. Vegans often rely on foods such as soy milk, soy yogurt, soy margarine, and soy- or rice-based "ice cream" to satisfy their desires for familiar favorites. However, these products are not available to all vegans, either because they are too expensive for some people's limited means or are not obtainable locally. As Jenny, a lacto-ovo-vegetarian for seven years, explained:

> I would love to find affordable alternatives to these cruelly produced foods, but have been thus far unable to do so.

> Many vegan alternatives are simply beyond my modest budget. And no food co-ops exist in my area. So for now I live with my guilt.

Third, some people are concerned about the complexity and difficulty of the transition. Many feel it would involve learning a whole new repertoire of recipes. Furthermore, many people invested a considerable amount of time in learning recipes based on cheese and eggs when they became lacto-ovo-vegetarians. Having to throw these recipes out and start from scratch learning how to prepare eggless and dairyless dishes is an onerous prospect. Some people anticipate difficulties in eating out, traveling, and socializing. These concerns are well-founded, and many people realistically anticipate the problems they would encounter.

In addition, some are concerned about the nutritional limitations of a diet based entirely on plant foods. As Drew, a computer programmer and vegetarian for two years, put it:

> We have not yet given up cheese, butter, and milk. We know we should. We know of the connection between the veal calf and the milk. We don't know if we will have the stamina to take that step, chiefly because we are afraid that it would force us, finally, to take cooking seriously. We'd have to study charts and concentrate endlessly on avoiding protein deficiency.

The above comment indicates that myths about the necessity of animal protein die hard. In fact, vegans have little difficulty in obtaining adequate protein, and conscientiously balancing plant foods for this purpose is not necessary (see our discussion in Chapter 1). Nevertheless, vegans should acquaint themselves with good plant sources of certain nutrients, such as iron, calcium, zinc, and riboflavin, and they should familiarize themselves with the B-12 controversy.

Finally, some people see value in veganism but talk themselves out of changing by rationalizing their consumption of dairy products and eggs. Mike, in a moment of self-insight, told us:

> As for becoming vegan, I would love to, but cheese and milk are a staple of my diet. I feel that the dairy cows are

treated well, for the most part. Yet, even as I say that, I realize I am clinging to the rationalization because of my weakness for cheese and milk. One day I will find the courage and strength to quit them.

THE CHANGE TO VEGANISM

As we pointed out in the previous section, a person's evolution as a vegetarian doesn't necessarily stop with abstinence from flesh. For many, the move to a completely plant-based diet—veganism—is a final step. And although lacto-ovo-vegetarians can think of good reasons for not becoming vegans, many eventually do. In our sample, 71 percent of vegans had spent a period of time as lacto-ovo- or lacto-vegetarians. (The other 29% went directly from being meat-eaters to vegans.) The average amount of time vegans spent as lacto-ovo- or lacto-vegetarians was four and one half years.

Is it difficult to become a vegan? Seventy-eight percent of vegans report having had difficulty with the transition. As noted above, only 27 percent of lacto-ovo-vegetarians describe giving up meat as difficult, so it appears that the change to veganism is relatively hard. This is not surprising, considering the pervasiveness of dairy products and eggs in the typical Western diet. Some vegans find it particularly difficult to give up old favorites, such as milk in coffee. Cheese is also greatly missed because it is a convenient filler for sandwiches and is used to top many dishes. Most processed foods, such as baked goods, contain dairy products or eggs, so vegans quickly learn that the number of items they can buy in their local supermarkets is greatly reduced. And, of course, eating out in most restaurants is difficult, if not impossible. Not surprisingly, many people feel that giving up dairy products and eggs is more problematic than giving up meat.

> Cheese was much harder to give up than meat because most of the meals I would make as a main course involved a lot of cheese, such as casseroles. Even vegetable type entrees always had a cheese sauce. And, when eating out,

> everything has cheese. It is very prevalent and hard to get away from. And I liked cheese as a topping on pasta.
>
> I don't think I ever craved meat but I really got into cheese. I was a big cheese person and it was really hard giving that up. I initially gave in to my cravings a lot but I would always ask myself if I wanted to support an industry that hurts animals, and the answer would be no.

As we noted earlier, most vegetarians, in spite of initial cravings, eventually come to find meat to be repugnant. A similar situation holds for vegans. Many who experience early difficulty in giving up cheese later have occasion to taste it again and are surprised to find that it isn't as nice as they remembered. Patrick, a university professor, described his experience with cheese:

> I hadn't eaten cheese in about six months. Then we went to an Italian restaurant and I had a pasta dish smothered in cheese. It had the texture of a coagulated clot of fat. And it smelled and tasted like a wet cow. I was disgusted.

As we noted earlier, many vegans complain that finding alternatives to dairy products is difficult in many parts of the country. The difficulty, however, is relative. For some long-term vegans, the 1980s are a vegan's paradise. In fact, the number of companies presently offering soy-based products has grown dramatically in the last few years. Laura, who has been vegan for 56 years, commented:

> Soy products are available everywhere now, salad bars abound, and vegetarian restaurants are plentiful. I feel privileged to be eating so bountifully and well with no effort at all.

Gwen, another long-term vegan, pointed out that vegan foods are becoming more popular and easier to obtain:

> Vegetarianism, and later veganism, are incredibly simple. Vegan food is limited only by one's imagination. And especially these days, with a staggering array of foods available, the choices of gourmet eating are endless. Ten years ago, foods like tofu, tempeh, miso, vegiburgers, soya ice cream,

> and frozen tofu desserts were unknown. Today, they are everywhere.

Not everyone experiences the transition to veganism similarly. Although many vegans find the transition to be difficult, others describe it as effortless. Often it is a rewarding and even pleasurable experience, in spite of occasional inconveniences. For example, Cynthia, her husband, and her children became vegan together. She described it as "a wonderful harmonious growing experience for us. There were no after-effects, cravings, or regrets of any kind." Lyndon, an English psychology student, had considered veganism for a long time but thought it would be too difficult. He had his expectations proven wrong by the following experience:

> In 1986 I gave up eggs and cheese for a period for economic reasons and then, when Chernobyl blew up, I gave up milk for health reasons. I found that I could manage without eggs, milk, and cheese and I even got to like soya milk, which I had never expected.

When all is said and done, however, there is no doubt that it is difficult to be a perfectly strict vegan; given the limited options that currently exist in our society, a certain amount of self-sacrifice is required. Nevertheless, it is possible to approach the vegan ideal, even if it is only imperfectly attained. Many of the people we spoke with were 95 to 99 percent vegan, with occasional liberties being taken in exceptional circumstances. For example, some "vegans" eat baked goods in restaurants, when traveling, or when staying with family, even though these might contain dairy products or eggs. Under these circumstances, they simply do the best they can, but with the realization that 100 percent consistency is probably not worth the extra effort. Such *practical veganism* is a realistic compromise for many vegetarians at this point in time.

Of course, as the number of vegans increases, the availability of alternatives to traditional dairy products will increase correspondingly. As an example of things to come, in Los Angeles—where trends often originate and spread eastward—a small chain of vegan fast-food restaurants is thriving. And recently, in San Diego, the first vegan pizza parlor opened. We believe that in the near future, an increasing number of vegetarians will opt for some form of veganism as the logical development of whatever motive led them to abstain from animal flesh in the first place.

We close with the following story from Stuart, an ethical vegetarian and journalist, which nicely encapsulates many of the trends described in this chapter: a gradual changeover in which meats are eliminated in stages, early vegetarian meals that can only be described as disgusting, the learning of vegetarian cooking skills and the delights of meatless cuisine, initial meat cravings that later turn to repugnance, and a successful transition to veganism in spite of minor inconveniences.

> I am a strict vegan. This is as radical a change as possible as I grew up hating vegetables and fruits and lived mainly on meat and desserts. First, I had to teach myself to eat vegetables, then I would eliminate meat. Initially, I ground up vegetables, mixed them with lots of breadcrumbs and eggs, baked the resultant gruel into a sort of soggy, flat loaf, and covered it all with mustard (which can cover any flavor). Then I reduced and soon eliminated the eggs. Eventually, I learned to try vegetables plain and slowly developed a real appreciaton for raw vegetables. Fruits were easier to learn to like. While this process was going on, I started eliminating meat from my diet, as follows: pork and veal went immediately; beef, gradually reduced portion-size until it was out of my diet; then chicken, same reduction technique down to zero; then eggs; then fish. Total time required for elimination of meat, poultry, eggs and fish was about three months. At this point I stayed lacto-vegetarian for about two years. The final break to a pure vegan diet seemed scary before I tried it, but turned out to be fairly easy. I also became a fair chef, and I think I make the best vegan chili and the best full-meal salads in the entire universe (excellent avocados are the key to the salad). I don't miss meat at all now; in fact, the sight and especially the smell of meat cooking has become offensive to me. Eliminating milk was more difficult, but only at breakfast time because I have to pour orange juice over my dry cereal (looks weird, tastes fair).

Clearly, if Stuart can become a vegan, anyone can.

Chapter 4

Implications of Vegetarianism for Personal Well-Being

As we have seen, many people become vegetarian because they anticipate benefits in the form of better health, personal growth, or an enhanced spiritual life. Do people really experience these rewards? Does vegetarianism make a difference? To answer these questions, we asked people about the ways in which they had changed since they became vegetarians. In framing our questions, we asked people to consider the health, psychological, ethical, spiritual, and sexual aspects of their lives.

We anticipated that people who stopped eating meat many years ago would find these questions difficult to answer. But for the great majority of vegetarians, the decision to give up meat is a major turning point in their lives. As such, it provides a marker that allows them to compare their feelings and experiences before and after. For many vegetarians, these changes are dramatic, obvious, and impossible to ignore. Consequently, most people in our sample, including long-term vegetarians, were able to respond to our questions without difficulty.

CHANGES IN PHYSICAL HEALTH

Eighty-four percent of people in our study report improvements in physical health after becoming vegetarian, 7 percent report decrements in health, and 9 percent report no change. Our figures are very similar to those reported in a 1987 *Vege-*

tarian Times reader poll; in their survey, 82.5 percent of readers said their health improved after they stopped eating meat, 1 percent said their health deteriorated, and 16 percent said there was no difference.[1] Overall, these results tell us that the great majority of people see themselves as being healthier since they became vegetarians. Furthermore, the fact that 7 percent of people in our study report decrements in health is deceptive, for about half of these people say their problems were temporary and that positive changes emerged later.

Is this just wishful thinking on the part of vegetarians? Probably not. As the American Dietetic Association pointed out in 1988, medical studies indicate that vegetarians have fewer problems with obesity, coronary heart disease, hypertension, diabetes, and several forms of cancer than do meat-eaters.[2] Researchers from the University of Texas recently conducted a study that supports this view. They found that twice as many nonvegetarians (27%) as vegetarians (12%) had been hospitalized within the previous five years.[3] The vegetarians in our sample may have exaggerated their level of health improvement somewhat, but their accounts are basically what one would expect on the basis of previous medical studies.

Of course, becoming a vegetarian is often only one aspect of a general improvement in lifestyle. At the same time that people stop eating meat, many also increase their consumption of fresh fruits, vegetables, and whole grain products; decrease their consumption of junk food, coffee, and alcohol; get more exercise; and adopt a more positive outlook on life. Given all of these potentially beneficial changes, it is difficult to disentangle the specific effects of a meatless diet. Indeed, it may be misleading to do so, for people's diets are often an expression of more general attitudes and lifestyle patterns. We should keep this total pattern of change in mind as we examine the improvements in health that people in our study report.

Positive Changes

The most common positive changes (and the percentage of people who report them) are: an increase in energy and stamina (31%), being sick less often—in particular, fewer colds and flu

(21%), the curing of a preexisting health problem (16%), better digestion and more regular bowel movements (10%), improved complexion, nails, hair, or teeth (8%), a weight problem that was brought under control (7%), and looking or feeling "younger" (7%). In addition, 26% report a general improvement in their physical well-being without mentioning any specific change. (These percentages add to more than the 84% reporting positive changes because some people mention more than one benefit.) One might note that these changes do not simply reflect a tendency for people to be sick less often, but to feel generally healthier. As such, they suggest a broad improvement in the daily quality of life.

Increased Energy

Nearly one out of every three vegetarians report an enhanced level of energy, stamina, and endurance, making this the most commonly mentioned health-related benefit. Many people who notice an improvement in energy are involved in sports or athletics. Not surprisingly, they find that giving up meat is associated with better performance. As Samuel told us:

> I'm an athlete. A lot of people look at me and they think vegetarians should be skinny, weak, and fragile. But I've run marathons, biathalons, triathalons, and ultra-distance events. I teach tennis. I have found that the vegetarian diet in no way limits your ability to be physical. If I'm in a long distance event, such as a 24 hour race, I've found the vegetarian diet is much easier on my system.

In addition to athletes, those who lead physically active lives also find a vegetarian diet to be beneficial. For example, shortly after becoming a vegetarian, Philip and a friend went on a bicycle trip from Southern California to Canada and back—a distance of several thousand miles. As Philip said, "Despite what meat-eaters say about a loss of strength, I found that a long distance bicycle tour and vegetarianism are compatible." Greg, a small-business owner, had a similar experience:

> I go for long bike rides and I never bog down for lack of energy. I do 40- to 50-mile rides, and I'm fine. I think it has

> a lot to do with diet. The foods vegetarians eat are easier to digest, so you're not bogged down by undigested food.

In a similar vein, others claim that being vegetarian helps them to cope with a busy lifestyle. Some feel that a meatless diet gives them a competitive edge in their line of work. Peter, an academic, made the following point:

> I have more energy now that I've stopped eating all animal products. This helps me to keep up with a hectic lifestyle of preparing lectures, teaching, conducting research, writing scientific papers, presenting papers at conventions, and keeping up with the literature in my area. Academia is highly competitive, and I feel that my diet helps me to maintain my productivity and to be successful in my career.

Even strict vegetarians—whom many think of as weak and emaciated from their diets based entirely on plant foods with no animal protein—often have physically demanding lifestyles. The comments below are from two natural hygienists, the first from Frank, a 58-year-old man, and the second from Constance, a 31-year-old woman:

> Physically, I am still very hale and hearty, continue to bicycle, doing anywhere from 30 to 50 miles on any given day, and continue to take long walks, go hiking and mountain climbing with members of the Appalachian Mountain Club, and never take public transportation when I can walk. I do not own or operate a motor vehicle and get as much outdoor exercise as is humanly possible.

> I lift weights at the local gym four times a week for one hour, plus I exercise every morning for one hour. Sometimes I get a short walk in the afternoons in too. During the weekends I enjoy hiking in the Santa Cruz mountains.

Most people believe that meat provides energy for hard physical work and exercise; to them, the high energy level of vegetarians would appear puzzling. However, it is not protein, but complex carbohydrates—such as pasta, bread, rice, and potatoes—that provide energy to the body.[4] The fact that vegetarians, compared with meat eaters, tend to consume a greater proportion of their daily calories in the form of complex carbohydrates could be a factor in their high levels of endurance. In addition, vegetarians tend to eat less fat than do meat-eaters. Research conducted by Judith Wurtman and her colleagues at the Massachusetts Institute of Technology indicates that fat takes a relatively long time to digest; consequently, after a high-fat meal, blood is diverted to the stomach and intestines and away from the brain. According to Wurtman, this can result in feelings of lethargy and drowsiness.[5] The low-fat diets of most vegetarians, therefore, should help them to avoid these low-energy states. Of course, vegetarians tend to be health-conscious people, and most keep their alcohol consumption down and get plenty of exercise. It is likely that a combination of these positive health factors contributes to the high energy levels experienced by many vegetarians.

Fewer Illnesses

As noted above, about one in five vegetarians claim to get sick less often since giving up meat. Most of these people say they get fewer colds and chest infections than they used to.

> The winter before giving up meat, we were plagued by colds, laryngitis, bronchitis, and other ailments. The winter after becoming vegetarian, my husband and I each suffered from one head cold, much less severe and bothersome than others we had [had] previously.
>
> I had a kidney transplant three years ago, so I'm on immune suppressant drugs. But in the past three years I've had the flu maybe once, and that is pretty rare because people on immune suppressants are highly susceptible to respiratory problems.

Is there any reason for believing that people really have fewer colds after they stop eating meat? A diet high in animal fat and cholesterol can inhibit the functioning of the immune defense system, leading to frequent illnesses.[6] In contrast, vegetarians eat plenty of fresh fruits and vegetables, and for this reason get sufficient quantities of vitamin C and other nutrients, thus strengthening their ability to fight off infection.

Vegetarians who do not consume dairy products may have an additional advantage, for some individuals—about one person in four—have allergic reactions to the protein in milk. These reactions can take the form of nasal stuffiness, runny nose, or other respiratory problems that mimic cold symptoms. People with milk allergies generally report fewer respiratory problems after eliminating dairy products from their diets.[7]

Preexisting Health Problems Improved

About one person in six finds that preexisting health problems improve or disappear after giving up flesh foods. In some cases, people are plagued with symptoms for years and turn to a vegetarian diet as a possible solution. Many are pleasantly surprised to find that this dietary change appears to bring the symptoms under control. The problems we heard of include allergies, asthma, chest pains, frequent headaches, arthritis, irritable bowel, hypoglycemia, gum disease, hemorrhoids, varicose veins, premenstrual syndrome, and glaucoma.

Toni, a writer, was a walking textbook of medical problems. Later, she adopted a well-balanced lacto-vegetarian diet that eliminated junk food and included a good deal of fresh fruits and vegetables. The resulting improvement in her health was marked:

> I was an avid meat-eater, raised on steaks on the grill, prime rib, hamburgers, hot dogs—the usual. I ate little or no vegetables or fruit. I had my tonsils and appendix out, bladder infections, mono, viral meningitis, and allergies. I also had chronic headaches and asthma. I was on muscle relaxers, antihistamines, and allergy shots when I got married. Soon afterward, I stopped eating meat. About the same time, I stopped eating most sweets and pop. A year later, I stopped eating eggs and dairy products. In the course of time, my health steadily improved. After four years, I have no more allergies, no asthma, no bladder infections, and virtually no headaches. My complexion also cleared up and my periods have regulated.

Sheila also suffered from poor health for many years. She found that a combination of fasting and a strict vegetarian diet based on the principles of natural hygiene alleviated her health problems:

> I have suffered from severe bronchial asthma from the time I was about 6 or 7. I was in and out of hospital, was receiving allergy shots, and was making numerous night trips to the emergency room for shots of adrenaline. By the age of 25, I had had it. I was on six types of medications, each of which I was taking three or four times daily, and I still couldn't breathe. I decided it was time to try something different. I went to a health sanctuary and fasted. I went off all my medication and after a while I found I could breathe clearly. As long as I stuck to the hygienic diet of fruits, raw vegetables, and seeds, I didn't have asthma. When I ate bread or dairy products, it returned. After this, I got progressively stronger.

It is possible that Sheila's bronchial problems were brought on by food allergies. Earlier, we pointed out how common dairy allergies are. In addition, some people are allergic to meat and animal fat or to the chemicals commonly found in them. Allergic reactions to plant foods can also occur, with wheat allergies being the most common. Sheila's problems were quite likely linked to foods that her natural hygienist diet avoids.

Food allergies often lead to health problems beginning in childhood. Unfortunately, the cause of these problems sometimes remains undiagnosed until adulthood. As Julie, a lacto-vegetarian of 10 years, told us:

> I've been sick all my life. I always had trouble at school. My IQ was higher than average but my concentration was poor. They took blood tests and I wasn't anemic and the doctors were totally confused. In those days they didn't know anything about hypogylcemia. They finally found out that all the chemicals and fat content in meat were making me very ill. My symptoms were quite severe. I was getting dizzy spells and blackouts.

After receiving medical advice, Julie eliminated all meat from her diet; shortly afterward, her problems disappeared.

Roxanne, an apartment manager, also discovered that she was allergic to substances found in meat. As in Julie's case, adopting a vegetarian diet led to a marked improvement in her condition:

> I had a severe allergy to two frequently used antibiotics, tetracycline and penicillin. These two drugs are used extensively on farm animals. Upon learning of this, I decided to stop consuming all meat to determine how much of a negative effect these foods were having on my severe asthma. Approximately two months after I had stopped eating meat, my condition dramatically improved to the point that I could completely eliminate the use of my steroid inhaler, plus reduce my use of the maintenance drug, theophylline, by two-thirds. The side effects of these drugs were unbearable. I would shake uncontrollably at any given time, and sometimes my voice would quaver, making me appear extremely nervous. It is a major relief to finally have control of my body.

In many cases, it is not clear whether people's chronic health problems are due to a meat or dairy allergy or to some other cause. The fact that health problems improve or disappear altogether after meat withdrawal might indicate an allergy, or it might simply reflect a general improvement in physical health associated with a new diet. Whatever the cause, respondents who are cured of their symptoms usually credit the vegetarian diet with having given them a new lease on life. As Roxanne put it, "Vegetarianism gave me my life back. Now I feel normal."

Goodbye to Constipation

One in ten people report fewer problems with constipation and more regular bowel movements. This is due to the high fiber content of most vegetarian diets, particularly ones that contain frequent servings of whole grains, legumes, fruits, and vegetables. Fiber, which remains undigested, contributes bulk to the stools and helps them to pass through the colon more easily. The typical American diet is low in fiber, and the presence of laxatives on so many bathroom shelves is a clear indication that chronic constipation is a fact of life in this country. Many people notice a marked change in the regularity of their bowel movements shortly after adopting a vegetarian diet:

> It was wonderful. This is embarrassing, but I don't mind saying it. I had a life-long problem with constipation which cleared up immediately. It was so dramatic and so obviously connected with giving up meat that I can't see it happened for any other reason.

Better Complexion, Hair, Nails, and Teeth

Some people mention improvements in hair or complexion. For example, Andy, a vegan for nine years, found that his severe acne cleared up shortly after he stopped eating dairy products. Peter, an amateur classical guitarist, experienced problems with the fingernails on his right hand constantly splitting and breaking. However, shortly after changing from a lacto-ovo-vegetarian to a vegan diet, he noticed that his fingernails became "hard as steel." A few respondents note cleaner teeth. Maria, a homemaker and vegetarian for 10 years, told us:

> I went to the dentist recently and he was surprised and pleased at how clean my teeth are. I explained our vegetarian whole grain diet, and he concurred that such high fiber food helps scrub the teeth and keep them clean.

Weight Loss

Obesity is relatively uncommon among vegetarians. This is due to the fact that most meats are high in calories, whereas fruits, vegetables, grains, and legumes are naturally low in calories. Studies confirm that vegetarians consume, on average, fewer calories than do meat-eaters. However, although plant foods are low in calories, they contain bulk which contributes to a feeling of fullness. Consequently, a diet based largely on plant foods leaves people feeling well-fed without contributing to obesity. Indeed, many vegetarians boast that they can eat as much as they like without putting on weight.

Weight loss is common when people stop eating meat. Half of the people in our sample lost weight during the transition to vegetarianism, and many vegans lost additional weight when they gave up dairy products. Our results are similar to those reported in a *Vegetarian Times* reader poll: Fifty-three percent of women and 54 percent of men claimed to have lost weight since adopting a vegetarian diet. In our study, for those who lost weight, the number of pounds ranged from 2 to 90 with a median value of 20. Mark, a cab driver, found that his weight problem improved when he stopped eating meat:

> I became a vegetarian in January of 1986, at which time I weighed 200 pounds. My weight as of July 1, 1987, was 171 pounds. I have a sweet tooth and rarely does a day go by that I don't eat plenty of sweets. But I'm still losing weight. When I ate meat, even though I exercised frequently, I stayed at exactly the same weight for five years.

Although weight loss is common, a few people report putting on weight after turning vegetarian. If one replaces the meat in one's diet with large servings of high-fat vegetarian foods, such as cheese, whole milk, and nuts, this is certainly a possibility. This occurs infrequently, however, because people tend to eat cheese and nuts in smaller quantities than they eat meat.

More Youthful?

A few people claim that their diets are related to their looking unusually young for their ages. For example, several vegetarians who were in their late 30s and early 40s said that people usually think they are about 10 years younger. Some people literally believe that giving up meat has caused them to age more slowly. Others say that being vegetarian makes them *feel* younger. Although a meatless diet is probably not the fountain of youth, having more energy and being slimmer might indeed cause some vegetarians to appear younger than their age.

In this context, it is relevant to note that in carrying out our research, we spoke with quite a few "older" people who were in good health, physically active, and young in outlook. This group included three women who had each been vegetarian for over 50 years; all led full and busy lives. Mildred told us about her daily routine:

> I do not accept the envious comment that I am so lucky to have an 82nd birthday coming up. I have never been hospi-

talized, carry no health insurance, never take an aspirin or a pain pill. It isn't good luck, but thought, planning, self-discipline, and common sense. My daily walk of two to four miles (depending on the weather), writing assignments, and correspondence keep me pleasantly occupied.

General Improvements in Health

As we noted earlier, giving up meat is often the first step leading to a health-promoting lifestyle. Vegetarianism causes some people to become more aware and knowledgeable about nutrition. It leads others to attend more closely to their bodies' needs; as a result, exercise levels are increased and alcohol and cigarettes are abandoned. Vegetarians are probably more aware than the average person that most of the serious health problems that plague our society are due to lifestyle, and as such, can be prevented.

I am certainly not a health-fitness fanatic, but I find myself more willing to exercise than I was in the past—which was not at all—and also more willing to turn down desserts—which was never. I think giving up meat has put me more in touch with my own responsibilities for my health.

Since I became committed to doing what I can for animal rights, I became committed also to living more fully and honestly. For that reason, I gave up drinking alcohol, which had become a problem in my life. The animal movement put me back in touch with nature, and now I much prefer the elation of a clear mind.

Health Problems

As noted above, 7 percent of people report a deterioration in health after adopting a vegetarian diet. Weakness, tiredness, light-headedness, and poor complexion are the problems mentioned most frequently. In about half these cases, however, problems clear up after the first few months. Some people describe this period as a "healing crisis."

After I adopted a macrobiotic diet, my mother thought I lost that twinkle in my eye. That's OK. My energy was a little

> weak for a while. There's a certain amount of toxins we have to release.
>
> The first month was rough. I experienced lightheadedness, pale skin color, and lack of energy. But on the positive side, my digestion improved, my sinuses cleared up, and I lost several inches off my waist.

Two people who were body builders—one male and one female—told us they experienced problems after giving up meat, in terms of both strength and ability to put on muscle mass. Both respondents, however, were in other ways active and in excellent health. Jim, a vegan who works in a food cooperative, told us:

> One thing I did notice. I was lifting weights and working out a lot before the transition. And I noticed after about a month that my strength was sapped. Even though I was eating a lot of tempeh and was getting a lot of protein, I definitely lost a huge amount of strength. Now my endurance is good, but I don't have as much strength as before.

A small number of people mention problems related to dietary deficiencies—the fear of many recent converts to vegetarianism. In these cases, the problems appear to have occurred because the people knew little about nutrition and were on inadequate "junk food vegetarian" diets. As we noted earlier, many people do not know what to cook after eliminating meat and wind up eating poor-quality foods for a period of time. In most cases, people eventually realize the problem and take steps to improve their diet.

> I had a terrible diet. I was living on french fries, Coke, and candy. I had no awareness. I came down with a number of health problems and I had a lot of depression. I'm sure it was linked.

Overall, reports of nutritional deficiencies are rare among vegetarians. This is encouraging, particularly in light of the fact that we spoke with so many vegans and others on relatively strict diets. In principle, long-term vegans should be at risk for developing Vitamin B-12 deficiency. Yet, we encountered no vegans who had experienced this problem. Of course, B-12 deficiencies can take 20 to 30 years to develop, so all the evidence is not yet in. Perhaps future research will one day determine if vegans are any more at risk of B-12 deficiencies than are other people.

No Change

Nine percent of people report no change in health or physical well-being after eliminating meat. In many of these cases, people are already in excellent physical health before modifying their diets, so there is little room for improvement. As Mary, a vegetarian of 19 years, commented:

> I can run circles around, work the pants off, and generally out-distance any one of my decaying-flesh-eating acquaintances—but I could when I ate flesh too. I've come to believe that as long as a human has food of any kind, he'll be all right. And the energy level is inherited.

Other people simply notice no difference. This is understandable, since there is no reason why vegetarianism should affect everyone in the same manner, particularly in light of the great diversity of diets to which vegetarians adhere. Some vegetarians feel that the health advantages of a meatless diet are overrated. Usually, these people are ethical vegetarians. For example, Robert, an animal rights activist, felt that there are no major health consequences of not eating meat. As he said, "The whole thing is a lot of fuss about something that is very trivial."

How Reliable Are People's Reports?

The accounts of vegetarians strongly support the notion that eliminating meat from one's diet results in a variety of beneficial changes in health and physical well-being. However, these accounts of positive changes are subject to a few limitations. First, when people are asked about events that happened in the past, their memories may be cloudy or in error on certain points.

Second, some people may exaggerate the benefits of vegetarianism to present a favorable picture of their own lifestyles. Finally, some may simply report what they expect to happen. In other words, if people expect to feel better after giving up meat, then they may "con themselves" into believing that they feel better even in the absence of any physical indications. (This is called the "placebo effect.")

One way of checking the degree of distortion in our results is to compare the level of health improvement reported by two groups of vegetarians: those who stop eating meat entirely for reasons of personal gain and those who stop eating meat entirely for ethical–social reasons. Since ethical–social vegetarians do not abstain from flesh because they anticipate health benefits, their expectations should not strongly influence their perceptions. Ethical vegetarians are also less likely than personal gain vegetarians to engage in other health-promoting behaviors. Indeed, some people who stop eating meat for ethical reasons become "junk food vegetarians"; to them, improvements in health are irrelevant. Consequently, ethical–social vegetarians will stick with their diets even if they do not experience improvements in health, whereas health-oriented people may return to eating meat if the benefits they anticipate are not forthcoming.

As it turns out, 91 percent of personal gain vegetarians report improvements in health compared with 71 percent of ethical–social vegetarians. The fact that the majority of ethical–social vegetarians also report health benefits suggests that improvements are the norm for most people and that the generally positive picture of vegetarian health is not overly exaggerated.

PSYCHOLOGICAL CHANGES

Vegetarians experience a variety of changes in feelings, outlook, and values after excluding meat from their diets. Overall, 89 percent of people report positive changes, 8 percent report negative changes, and 3 percent report no change. It is noteworthy that such a large proportion of people experience positive outcomes; although the physical health benefits of a meatless diet have been frequently discussed, much less has been said about possible psychological benefits. Yet, they appear to be as common as the physical ones.

Positive Changes

The most commonly reported changes include: an enhanced sense of morality and responsibility (21%), feeling more peaceful and less aggressive (19%), an increase in self-esteem (19%), a decrease in feelings of guilt (17%), an expanded awareness of nature and one's place in it (16%), an increase in feelings of compassion (12%), an increase in happiness and general sense of well-being (12%), an increase in emotional stability (7%), greater mental clarity and ability to concentrate (6%), and enhanced willpower (6%). (These percentages add to more than the 89% reporting positive changes because some people reported more than one type of change.)

About one in five vegetarians refer to changes in their sense of morality. Many people say that vegetarianism has given them a new moral purpose and something to believe in. For these individuals, every meal is an opportunity to demonstrate their commitment to their ideals. And because they feel that what they are doing is ethically correct, most experience a deep sense of satisfaction. As one would expect, most of these people are ethical vegetarians.

> My life has improved greatly for finally having something bigger than myself. Vegetarianism and animal rights is where my heart has always belonged.

> The big benefit is that I feel as comfortable as I can with my lifestyle. I feel that I'm putting into practice what I believe to be ethically right and I feel really, really positive about it.

In the past, religion, the extended family, and the local neighborhood provided a sense of tradition and continuity with the past. But in a materialistic era of consumerism, family instability, and the anonymity of large cities, many people have trouble finding a moral center to their lives. Consequently, the sense of purpose provided by vegetarianism is extremely important to some people. For them, it provides a general philosophy of life that gives meaning to day-to-day events. Martha, a homemaker, found that vegetarianism gave her life a new ethical direction:

> The most important aspect of vegetarianism to me is the moral and spiritual one. I had no religious guidance of any kind while I was growing up. My parents did not attend church, and as far as I can remember, never once gave me any direction, any code of ethics, any moral foundation to build a life on. I had always felt "cast adrift" with no mooring. Conformity was the only lesson I ever learned. This is what I like about vegetarianism; it has opened up a whole ethical life for me. I can live this philosophy. It gives me something concrete to do, ethically, every day.

For a few individuals, vegetarianism becomes the central focus of their lives. As Mike, a high school teacher, stated:

> I feel that my entire life, my existence on the planet, my very soul has been immeasurably improved and upgraded since that amazing moment my eyes were opened to the purity and rightness of a vegetarian lifestyle. If I never amount to anything else in life, at least I've lived as a protector and benefactor of the beasts.

Many people believe that abstaining from meat makes a person peaceful. Consistent with this notion, almost one in five vegetarians report feeling less aggressive since rejecting meat. This is not to be confused, however, with feeling weak or lethargic, as our earlier discussion of health improvements demonstrated. As Philip said, "I feel a lot more peaceful now, more relaxed, and calmer. I'm not as hot-headed as I used to be. But I can still play a mean game of tennis, which surprises some people."

Why should a vegetarian diet make people feel less aggressive? One answer is based on recent findings in human neurophysiology. Studies have shown that certain chemicals, referred to as "neurotransmitters," act to relay messages in the brain. One particular chemical, serotonin, is associated with feelings of lowered tension and relaxation. Eating carbohydrates such as legumes, whole grain products, and vegetables causes the brain to increase its uptake of tryptophan, an amino acid. This, in turn, causes the brain to produce serotonin.[8] Because vegetarians generally replace the calories in their diets from meat with carbohydrates, it is probable that their brains manufacture relatively high levels of this neurotransmitter. This would account for their tendency to report feeling calm and peaceful much of the time.

Food allergies could also be a factor. Allergies to certain foods, such as milk, can result in feelings of irritability and anxiety. People with dairy allergies could find that their mood improves a good deal when they become strict vegetarians.[9]

Another common reaction, reported by almost one in five vegetarians, is to feel better about oneself. Many people take a good deal of pride in the fact that they are able to give up eating meat. As we noted earlier, becoming a vegetarian is difficult for many people; not only are cravings for meat sometimes a problem, but friends and family members are often unsupportive (as we discuss later). Because vegetarians are able to change in spite of these handicaps, and because they believe in the ethical correctness of their behavior, an increase in self-esteem is the result.

> I can remember when I first became aware of the cruelty to animals. The first time I went to the store to buy cruelty-free products I just felt so good to know that I was making a statement by doing that. I feel very good about myself.
>
> When I gave up meat I felt like less of a savage. I used to binge on meat. I would feel like I was a lion tearing up flesh. And when I gave it up I felt much better about myself and thought, "Well, at least I'm not a savage animal." I felt a lot more civilized.

About one in six vegetarians refer to a decreased sense of guilt. Feelings of guilt are common in many people's minds during the time preceding their change to vegetarianism. After learning about the grim realities of factory farming, it is difficult for many to feel good about their diets and behavior. Some individuals are able to rationalize their continued consumption of meat, but for those who face the issue squarely, a change in behavior is the only ethically correct choice. Under these circumstances, giving up meat is like having a weight lifted from one's back. People experience a clear conscience after becoming vegetarians and no longer have to apologize to themselves—or to others—for what they eat.

> Because I look at an animal and feel love rather than hunger, I am able to look at myself and feel love rather than guilt.
>
> At long last I feel spiritually satisfied. I do not have the death and suffering of other nonhuman animals on my conscience.

Along these lines, Bruce told us a story about how becoming a vegetarian changed his feelings toward animals:

> A friend of mine told me that one of the benefits of no longer eating animals is that they become your friends. She said that I could now walk through a field of cows and tell them that I no longer ate them and was their friend. I tried it shortly after becoming vegetarian, and although it seemed a bit silly at the time, even though I was alone, it did make me feel good to say it out loud.

An "increase in awareness" is mentioned by about one in six respondents. This includes a number of related changes: an expanded sensitivity to nature and animals, a clearer understanding of one's place in the world, and being more awake to objectionable practices that are carried out in the world. This change in awareness often involves an independent and critical view of our society. Martha, for example, felt that becoming a vegetarian had expanded her understanding in several ways:

> So many billions of animals are slaughtered for those sleepwalking, thoughtless humans. And I used to be one. I'm so glad I'm not one anymore. I feel more awake and alive than ever. And now I find myself looking for other blind spots in my thinking. I used to wonder how Hitler could have come to power and done all those atrocious things. Now I know. He succeeded because the vast majority of us don't think

> critically. We don't want to know. "Don't bother me" is the attitude.

Another commonly reported psychological change involves increased feelings of compassion. Some say that being vegetarian has led them to have more sympathy and concern for animals. Interestingly, vegans are more likely than lacto-ovo-vegetarians to report this change. Michael, a medical doctor, explained how becoming a strict vegetarian had changed his feelings:

> The years since my "quantum leap" into vegan nutrition for medical and health reasons have seen my personal evolution as an ethical vegan. My awareness has now grown to include nonviolent living principles in all aspects of my daily life, for example, clothing choices, consumer goods, gentleness in thought and action, and concern for the plight of all the animals who share our planet and suffer at the hands of man.

Others add that their feelings of compassion have grown to include humans as well. Some critics argue that ethical vegetarians are more concerned with animals than they are with people. But for many, becoming vegetarian involves an expansion of one's circle of compassion to include all living things. As one person put it, "Being a vegetarian makes me feel a gentleness towards all life, human and nonhuman alike."

About one in ten vegetarians claim that their diets help them to maintain their emotional stability. They feel that since giving up meat, they are less subject to mood fluctuations and more in control of their emotions. Many also believe that their diets help them to cope effectively with frustration or stress. One person described the change this way: "I think I have a better grip on my emotions than I used to. I'm not as moody as I used to be. If I'm angry, it is just anger and not a lingering thing."

These changes may be related to the effects of a low-fat diet based on complex carbohydrates. Carbohydrate consumption, as we noted earlier, causes the brain to produce serotonin, a neurotransmitter associated with feelings of relaxation. As such, a low-fat vegetarian diet is well-suited for people who must deal with high levels of everyday stress. The "emotional stability" effect may also be due to general improvements in health brought about by changes in diet and other lifestyle factors.

Another advantage that some people cite is an increase in mental clarity, alertness, and the ability to concentrate.

> One of the most important advantages of a total vegetarian diet is the capability to focus fully on one thing at a time and to experience full clarity of thought and purpose.

> When I gave up meat I didn't notice any difference. But after giving up cheese I felt a lot clearer in the head. I could think better. I felt a lot less sluggish and I had more energy. I wasn't as tired all the time—both physically and mentally.

A few even claimed an increase in intelligence. As one person stated, "Since becoming vegetarian, my IQ has gone up 20 points." Enhanced intellectual ability was also noted by a student who became vegetarian during her last year at college. As she said, "My grades in college really climbed after I became a vegan. During the last semester, I got all As—a first in a lifetime occurrence." Although interesting, we know of no direct evidence for increased intelligence. However, physical health is correlated with intelligence; for example, deteriorating health, particularly in old age, is associated with a decline in measured intelligence. So it is possible that a change to a health-promoting vegetarian lifestyle, particularly among people who are not living up to their full intellectual potential, could lead to an increase in mental performance.

Finally, some people mention an increase in will power and self-control. Becoming a vegetarian is a challenging experience. For those who succeed, eliminating meat from one's diet can serve as a good lesson in how to control other aspects of behavior. And success in one major undertaking increases people's confidence that they can change other aspects of their lives. As one person said:

> My becoming a vegetarian has benefited me in that I have a realization of my own will power and inner strength. I am

> much more disciplined in other areas of my life now as a result of my dietary restrictions.

Negative Changes

The material presented above indicates that the great majority of people experience positive psychological outcomes after they stop eating meat. Unfortunately, there is a dark side to this picture, with some people experiencing psychological problems. In almost all cases, these people are ethical vegetarians who are involved in the animal rights movement. Their distress is not caused by the diet itself, but by their awareness of the massive scale of slaughter and suffering caused to animals—an awareness that is accentuated by living as a vegetarian. These negative feelings take the form of depression, anger, bitterness, and hopelessness. Some people become obsessed with thoughts of cruelty to animals and find it difficult to think of anything else.

> I was beset by depression and outrage and an overwhelming sense of helplessness. I couldn't sleep at night thinking of the pain laboratory animals were enduring. That was four years ago, and while I've long since lost the overwhelming depression, there are moments when I can hardly stand to be in the human species because of its cruelty toward all life.

> The level of despair regarding animal torture I have felt on occasion is very intense and sometimes gets interpreted as bitterness. There have been times when my cling to life has been very tentative at best. I often resent being called a human being and having to call others around me brother. My sense of shame for their deeds in the name of science, health, and every other excuse reaches great depths. The spiritual foundation of our world is very weak—not built on ideals or love for anyone but self.

Some ethical vegetarians do not have any friends or family who share their concerns about animals. And because they feel so strongly about their beliefs, they find it difficult to socialize with meat-eaters, particularly since so many social activities revolve around food. Consequently, they experience loneliness and a sense of social isolation. As one person said, "It is extremely depressing that no one else believes in my values. This is emotionally and spiritually disturbing to me." Another person was more bitter: "I feel isolated from the rest of humanity because it's hard not to feel disgust at most people's attitudes."

We noted above that many people feel more peaceful and less aggressive after giving up meat. In contrast, others feel continuing anger at those who exploit animals, and this anger is sometimes expressed in feelings of aggression. As Andy, a vegan and animal rights activist, put it:

> In 1979 I visited a factory hog farm. It was the worst, most depressing thing I'd seen in my life. I felt like killing the owner and every ignorant human breezing by in their cars. When I saw a video on vivisection, it dredged up all my old feelings toward researchers: "Let's get our guns and kill those worthless bastards."

Andy's strong feelings may surprise some people. However, once there is an acceptance of the idea that people should extend compassion to all animals, the knowledge that we cause suffering to cows, pigs, sheep, and chickens on a massive scale has a powerful impact. To many ethical vegetarians, modern methods of factory farming are the moral equivalent of slavery or concentration camps. Given these strong feelings, it is not surprising that a small number of animal rights activists have formed direct action groups to "rescue" farm animals from certain death. Although members of these groups are often motivated by feelings of anger as well as compassion, most have taken a pledge of nonviolence—a position consistent with the vegetarian ideal.

Sometimes becoming an ethical vegetarian leads to a questioning of the world as a secure and benign place. Ken, a packager and vegetarian for two years, felt overwhelmed by the enormity of animal suffering in the world:

> I feel melancholic most of the time because most people seem unaware of the extent to which the human species has an adverse effect on the biosphere. I am also sad because I do not know why the force(s) that created space and

> matter would create a world where sentient beings are consumed by other sentient beings.

For some ethical vegetarians, humankind's exploitation of animals becomes an obsession and they find it difficult to avoid dwelling continually on painful thoughts. This can lead to "burnout," or worse, to psychological breakdowns from which people need professional help, and time, to recover. Carla, a nurse, described her experience:

> Shortly after becoming a vegetarian, I saw an old film of an elephant being electrocuted to see how many volts it took. I cried and was so depressed at the cruelty that it affected me for several days. Even when I would see a dead animal in the road, I wouldn't go that way again for a week. I couldn't get the thoughts of torture or death of animals out of my mind. I began seeing a psychologist. Over a two year period he helped me a great deal. I finally felt it was OK to be sensitive and unique. I still don't know why animals are so important to me, but I can cope with it now.

Some people dwell almost exclusively on how bad things are, but others report mixed outcomes: Although they feel sad or angry at the slaughter of animals, they are able to take pride in the fact that they are doing something positive by refusing to eat flesh. Many also avoid leather and make a point of purchasing cruelty-free household products and cosmetics. These actions give people a sense that they are no longer contributing to animal suffering, and that they are working toward an eventual solution to the problem. Laura, a marriage guidance counselor and recent convert to vegetarianism, felt this way:

> My brother always counselled me that as bad as I feel about these issues, the road to feeling better is to do something rather than try to avoid thinking about it. And he's right. I do feel much better about myself now that animals aren't dying just because I like the taste of their flesh.

The attitude expressed in the above quotation reflects a good strategy for coping with the unpleasant aspects of our culture's treatment of animals. Anger is destructive if it is turned inward toward the self, but it can be productive if it motivates behavior directed at bringing about social change. When one feels depressed, one should think, and do, something positive—not ruminate on how awful things appear to be. Many vegetarians take pride in the fact that their consumer choices contribute every day to the eradication of factory farming.

SPIRITUAL CHANGES

It is widely perceived that vegetarians are more "spiritual" than meat-eaters. Is there any truth in this notion? A previous study of vegetarians conducted by researchers at the University of Texas found that vegetarians are *less* likely than nonvegetarians to attend church or claim a religious affiliation.[10] Nevertheless, in our sample, more than one out of four vegetarians mention that changes in spiritual feelings occurred after they stopped eating flesh. Some of these people are religious vegetarians who adopt a meatless diet as part of their conversion to a new religion. Others are people with nonreligious motives who discover unanticipated spiritual implications of their new lifestyles. Of those who report changes, the great majority claim to feel more, rather than less, spiritual.

On the positive side, many people say that they feel closer to God since they stopped eating flesh. In most cases, this is because they no longer feel responsible for the killing of animals; this leaves them feeling peaceful and in harmony with both nature and God. A few people go as far as to describe the transition to vegetarianism as a spiritual experience:

> I felt more in harmony with the natural world and with the community of all living creatures. I felt closer to what Albert Schweitzer called our "spiritual relationship with the universe."

> My spiritual growth has been enormous in the past 18 years. I am much more aware of God now that I am helping Him instead of eating the creatures He created.

> When I became a vegan, I learned a new understanding of God—the first true spiritual experience I ever had. I real-

> ized then that God uses vegetarianism as an evolutionary litmus test.

Some say that their view of religion and God has become more positive since they stopped eating meat. For example, one person stated, "My concept of God has changed from One who is wrathful to a God who has made a wonderful, beautiful planet filled with lovable creatures." Others note that the transition to vegetarianism has led them to become more interested in religion. Many begin to read religious materials and think more about religious philosophy after giving up meat. As Constance, a natural hygienist, said:

> When I started living according to natural laws, I felt closer to God than I ever had in my life. I wanted to be pure in body, mind, and soul. I started reading inspirational material from all religions and traditions. It all spoke to me and I was cleansing on every level.

Most people find that vegetarianism complements their earlier religious views, and many are able to incorporate vegetarian themes into their belief systems. Stan, a journalist and vegan, had an unusual view on the relation between his diet and his religious beliefs:

> My faith is a mix of Christianity and primitive animism (belief that natural objects and forces have spirits). Vegetarianism is consistent with both views. The ministry of Jesus seems so oriented toward life and health and toward mercy that I must regard the incarnate God as a vegan, notwithstanding a few uncharacteristic scriptural passages which don't bother me, since my faith is in God, not in Biblical inaccuracy. And of course, in the animist view, it is wrong to kill any living creature needlessly, or to rape the planet. In sum, vegetarianism has strengthened and complemented my spiritual awakening and awareness.

In contrast, some vegetarians become *less* religious after changing their diets. In almost all cases, these people are ethical vegetarians. Their growing awareness of the massive suffering of animals in modern factory farms and laboratories leads them to question their former beliefs about God and religion. For them, the suffering of animals is inconsistent with a view of God as good or kind.

> Since finding out about the tortures inflicted on animals in laboratories, I am unsure whether to believe in a god or not. I know that no decent god would let something so unspeakable continue. I prefer to believe there is no God.
>
> I find it very difficult to find a place in any religious community due to my beliefs. For me, concern for all living beings is a spiritual issue. However, in most organized religions, I found that spiritual concern for others rarely goes beyond other humans. This I found disturbing. Personally, I can't believe that a benevolent God would create living, feeling creatures only to be eaten or used in other cruel ways by humans.

One person who felt this way was an ex-minister who later became an animal rights supporter. After rejecting his former beliefs, he became a member of American Atheists and the Freedom from Religion Foundation. His views about religion are particularly bitter, as his comments illustrate:

> I became a minister in 1974, but one interesting side effect of my involvement with animal rights has been a change of thinking regarding God. How can anyone love a God who enjoys animal sacrifice? This is the first thing Noah did after the flood. Leviticus 1 tells you how to rip animals apart as sacrifices. It's disgusting. God is not on our side. He gave fur coats to Adam and Eve to replace the fig leaves they were wearing. God accepted Abel's dead lambs, but not Cain's vegetables. God killed most animals with the big flood he created in order to kill the men, women, and children he didn't like. There are many examples of animal cruelty in the Bible, and intelligent people must conclude that such an evil God just cannot exist. If this God does exist, then the sensible alternative is to join Satan and try to overthrow him so that the animal abuse will stop.

Although spiritual changes are not uncommon, most people feel that vegetarianism has few implications for religion. Some believe that abstaining from meat has a potentially useful part to play in one's spiritual development, but vegetarianism alone is by no means a guarantee of a "higher" existence. Jack, a lacto-ovo-vegetarian for 15 years, saw himself as a spiritual seeker. Yet, he felt that the religious benefits of vegetarianism have been overrated:

> I am well aware that many higher-consciousness type groups teach that the vegetarian diet automatically makes one more spiritual, and, while I would guess there is some tendency to lead this way, the transformation is not at all automatic or inevitable. It may be a prerequisite, but is not a guarantee. I have found there is a whole lot more to this "higher path" than just the bean sprouts and tofu. It would be great if it was that easy and mechanical.

Clearly, the relation between vegetarianism and religion is an issue on which vegetarians differ a great deal.

SEXUAL CHANGES

Meat-eaters, as we all know, sometimes use oysters or exotic meats as aphrodisiacs. This might appear to leave vegetarians without any suitable recourse. However, as one person informed us, vegetarians use other vegetarians as aphrodisiacs. We were curious to know if becoming vegetarian has any implications for people's sexual urges, feelings, or behavior. As it turns out, the majority of people do not report any changes. But of those who do, 62 percent claim that their sex lives have improved.

We noted above that a common physical change is for people to experience an increase in their level of energy and endurance after eliminating meat from their diets. Not surprisingly, these enhanced capabilities are sometimes said to yield certain benefits in the bedroom:

> I feel healthier and have more energy and vitality. And this adds to my positive feelings about sex.

> This diet has made me feel sexier since I am thinner and have almost unlimited sexual energy. I have clear skin that is virtually wrinkle-free, even at age 35.

As the woman above noted, losing unwanted body fat can enhance one's sex appeal. Another person put it this way, "Before becoming vegetarian I was fat and unappealing. Now I'm lean in the sunshine and have a great love life." Certainly, in our culture, slimness is seen as a characteristic of physically attractive people. It is not surprising, therefore, that people who lose unnecessary body fat after adopting a vegetarian diet should find that their love lives improve. For one person, however, the loss of body fat led to a minor setback:

> Becoming a vegetarian reduced my body fat and gave me a leaner appearance, which is OK, except I do miss being two bra sizes larger. My husband misses it too, although, fortunately, he is a leg man and prefers small breasts to large ones. But although they are in hiding now, they'll meet the challenge if called upon.

For some, an improvement in sexual relations leads to more intimate and better-quality personal relationships with lovers and spouses. As one person said, "My sexual life? It's healthier, more spiritual, closer, and more committed." Another person put it this way: "My sex life is better because I have a better understanding of love than I ever had before becoming a vegan."

Some vegetarians say they couldn't imagine making love with someone who eats meat. Fellow vegetarians, it seems, are perceived as being more attractive, and sexier, than meat-eaters. As one woman told us, "I find my husband more sexually appealing knowing that he is not a vessel full of decaying carcasses."

Although an improved sex life is the most commonly noted outcome, some people feel that becoming vegetarian leads to a decrease in their level of sexual feelings. This response is given by 38 percent of people who report a change, but is particularly likely to be mentioned by natural hygienists. Often, this decline in sexual interest is said to occur when fasting or when eating a diet based entirely on raw foods.

> Since my fasts, I've had absolutely no sex drive. Before that, it was insatiable, due, I believe, to all the stimulants I was on.

> The purer one's diet, the less desire for sex. So it is absent when fasting. Eating cooked foods and animal products increases it.

When people do report a decrease in sexual feelings, however, it is generally viewed as a desirable outcome. These people place a high value on self-control, and less intense sexual urges are part of their desire for ascetic purity. The following comments, by a man and woman, respectively, illustrate this perspective:

> Since becoming vegetarian I've had a loss of sex drive, which is fine. Sexual energy can be better spent on other purposes.
>
> I no longer feel any strong sexual impulses, and believe me, I don't miss them. Life is much simpler when you don't feel the need to impress the opposite sex.

So, although some people's sex drive goes up after they stop eating meat and others' goes down, everyone seems to be satisfied.

EVALUATION OF FORMER SELF

Before finishing this chapter on personal changes, we examine people's views on their former lives as meat-eaters. Given that most people change in a variety of ways after becoming vegetarian, we were curious to know how people feel about their earlier selves. Would they feel remorse? Would they be ashamed of their previous behavior? Or would they accept it as a necessary part of their development?

We came across examples of these views—and some others that we did not expect. For one thing, we discovered that a large number of people had wanted to be vegetarians for years before they stopped eating meat. In many cases, these people had thought about being vegetarians since the time they were children, but had never acted on their feelings because of the constraints of living at home with parents. When these people grew up and left home, they generally did not become vegetarians immediately; they often took several years to get around to making the change. But the desire to be a vegetarian was always there. The following two stories, the first by a woman and the second by a man, illustrate this pattern:

> One day at about age 10, I saw uncooked chicken. It finally dawned on me that it was once alive like me. It ate, slept, and walked like me. I became very peculiar about my eating meat. It had to be very well done and swallowed down with bread or a vegetable. I objected to the idea of animals being slaughtered, but it wasn't until age 27 that I began living by that belief.

> When I was six or seven, I remember eating a steak and all the times I'd been told where meat comes from finally sank in. I remember asking, "You mean this used to be part of a cow that was walking around in a field?" I also remember saying I didn't think it was right to cut off part of an animal and eat it. It hadn't dawned on me yet that they killed the whole animal. I didn't want anything to do with the whole idea, but my parents assured me that I would die if I didn't eat meat.

These cases indicate that "meat insight" experiences, as we described earlier, can occur to young children as well as adults. Sometimes these insights occur unexpectedly, for no apparent reason, but they are usually generated by particular events. In Patty's case, this occurred when her father brought home the carcass of a deer he had shot:

> My father loved to hunt. I remember as a very young child, he brought home a deer and hung it upside down in the back yard. I went out and started petting it and crying because my father had killed this beautiful creature. How could anyone be so cruel—especially my own father? I then realized the deer meant meat on the table. I refused to eat any meat for about two weeks until I figured that deer meat was gone.

In a few cases, early experiences in which a close bond was formed with an animal generated a childhood revulsion to meat-eating. Barbara, a 26-year-old writer and lacto-ovo-vegetarian for eight years, told us the following story:

> When I was six years old, our family had a pet pig, and that's when I first began to realize the horror of eating meat—to make the connection between the pork chops and my wonderful pet "Pig-Pig." My mother reassured me that eating meat was simply the law of the jungle and what "God meant us to do." So I accepted it for the next several years, although feeling deep inside that it wasn't right.

Marcia, a 60-year-old homemaker and a lacto-ovo-vegetarian for 12 years, had a similar story to tell. She was raised on a farm in Canada, but her parents died when she was seven. Later she found solace in the company of the farm animals and spent most of her free time with the baby pigs (her favorites), calves, and chickens. These close relationships left a lasting impression on her. As she said, "I think this was the foundation for my decision, many years later, to become a vegetarian."

Lorie's father had been a butcher, and she recalled sad and eerie feelings from her childhood associated with her father's employment. Her experiences made her acutely aware of the death of animals, and this led her to consider vegetarianism later in life:

> I remember when my Dad had his butcher shop. We used to go down there and work with him. I used to come home and feel really irritated and I never knew why. But now I know. It was the vibrations. It was death. I also remember a meat-packing place. He used to take us there to pick up the beef. And it could have been the middle of summer in 90 degree heat, but it still felt cold. The coldness was the death that I was sensing. I could feel the death and I could smell it too. Sometimes I go to a grocery store and the odor comes back and the memory comes back of that time.

Others strongly disliked the taste or texture of meat as children and couldn't wait to stop eating it. These people look back to their period as meat-eaters with feelings of disgust. John, a produce manager for a natural food store, was one of these people:

> Meat was always the last thing I ever wanted to eat. I always liked the mashed potatoes and the vegetables. I grew up in a typical American family and that meant meat, po-

> tatoes, and vegetables. If we had fried chicken, I only liked the crispy stuff on the outside. If you bit into it, there were the veins, the arteries, and tendons. I definitely didn't like it. I don't blame my parents because they were brought up that way themselves. But it was forced on me.

These early experiences are predisposing factors to vegetarianism in later life. People who report these experiences go through a long period of discomfort and uneasiness as meat-eaters. For them, eating meat is something that has to be endured until circumstances are more favorable to making a change.

Another common pattern is fot people to realize that they had been duped—tricked by the meat industry and others into believing that meat is something other than an animal corpse. Of course, our cultural beliefs and practices are for the most part unconscious, and we rarely think about or question them. Our view of meat is no exception. Nevertheless, many people see themselves as having been extremely ignorant; many want to "kick themselves" for not having caught on earlier to the cruel hoax.

> I only wish I had come to the realization earlier in my life. I guess it's partly a matter of education. As soon as I was aware that the stuff that comes wrapped in plastic at the grocery store didn't always look like that, I got off it real quick. But I'm amazed at how long it took for me to put that together. I was into my 30s before I figured it out, and that's pretty sad.

Many children have a difficult time comprehending where meat comes from. Although it is not difficult to associate the tomato on the vine with the tomato in the salad, the relation between the cow in the field and the hamburger on one's plate is harder to grasp. Andy recalled his elaborate, although mistaken, childhood views about meat. His story illustrates the complex reasoning some children use in order to explain the mystery of meat:

> When I was small, I thought that cows laid meat like chickens do eggs. In a way, I thought that meat had some-

> thing to do with dung. Possibly, dung was processed into something we could eat. I also thought that hot dogs came out of pigs just like they look in the supermarket. When I hear kids ask, "Where does it come from?," and hear an adult say, "From a cow," nothing at all is cleared up. Maybe some adults think kids understand. Adults generally don't say, "Meat is the cow, a dead cow, and it was killed for you to eat." I couldn't imagine that animals were killed to eat. Later, with more awareness, I thought that these animals died natural deaths in the fields and we simply took their bodies.

Others were aware that meat was animal flesh, but believed that meat consumption is necessary, natural, or even humane. Glenda, a primary school teacher, explained how she had avoided the full implications of her beliefs for years:

> I had sympathized with the animal situation for a long time, but I guess I had justified it to myself, and this is why I never became vegetarian for moral reasons. I justified it in my own mind by thinking, "Man has been a hunter and fisher for food for years, and he always will be, regardless of whether I become a vegetarian or not."

Many people are disgusted with themselves for having taken such a long time to see the truth. For example, Brenda, an ethical vegetarian for five years, was critical of her former attitudes. As she said, "I was living in a dream world. I was indoctrinated into believing that the animals I was eating were not being hurt. My God, how could I have been so stupid."

Overall, regardless of how people evaluate their previous lives as meat-eaters, most regret that they waited so long to make the transition. It seems that if one is ever going to start, it is better to start now than later. As one person told us, "Every person is only one meal away from being a vegetarian."

SUMMARY

The great majority of people report positive changes after adopting a vegetarian diet. These include improvements in health and physical well-being as well as better psychological functioning and self-esteem. Many people also report that giving up meat has improved their sex lives, and others report that being vegetarian has increased their spiritual awareness. Clearly, people gain a lot when they become vegetarian. Although these positive trends are encouraging, one qualification is in order: A small minority of people experience health or psychological problems after adopting a vegetarian diet. Their experiences serve as a reminder that vegetarianism is not a universal cure-all, and that the road to a better lifestyle is sometimes rocky. We believe that many of these problems are unnecessary, and later we discuss ways of avoiding them.

Chapter 5

The Vegetarian Lifestyle

Being a vegetarian involves more than simply not eating meat. Most people don't realize the extent to which their diets are linked to other aspects of their lifestyles. But when people become vegetarians, they set off a chain reaction that affects numerous areas of their everyday lives. Some aspects of the vegetarian lifestyle vary depending on one's motives for abstaining from meat and the particular diet one follows. Nevertheless, regardless of one's motives or the types of food one eats, living as a vegetarian leads to a set of shared prospects and problems.

SO WHAT DO YOU EAT IF YOU DON'T EAT MEAT?

Meat-eaters often wonder what vegetarians manage to find to eat; many have the misconception that vegetarians live mainly on lettuce and raw carrots. Not surprisingly, people raised on meat-centered diets assume that a meal without flesh is incomplete. Perhaps more surprising is the fact that many novice vegetarians share the view that meatless meals are bland and boring. As we noted earlier, many people, when first excluding flesh from their diets, are not well prepared and don't know what to cook. As a result, their limited diets confirm the worst expectations of meat-eaters.

However, most people eventually discover the rich variety of plant foods that are commonly available. There are literally scores of different types of vegetables, grains, legumes, nuts, seeds, and fruits from which to build meals. In contrast, flesh-eaters must choose from cow, pig, chicken, sheep, turkey, and fish. Clearly, diversity exists in the plant kingdom—not in the realm of flesh foods. Consequently, most vegetarians do not view their diets as imposing onerous restrictions; instead, they find that vegetarianism opens up their eyes to a variety of new possibilities. Many discover that meatless versions of old favorites are even more delicious than the originals. Bill, a printer, told us how his early expectations of a bland meatless diet proved to be incorrect:

> My wife led the way and she dealt with the cooking. I thought I would miss meat but she brought in substitutes: tempeh, tofu, and things like that. I was surprised that the dishes could be as good, if not better, than the dishes made with meat.

Although initially experiencing some difficulty, many individuals discover that they enjoy the challenge offered by vegetarian cooking. Becoming a vegetarian requires learning a new set of skills, and many people gain a sense of accomplishment from discovering how to cook with new ingredients and mastering new dishes. Some people who have never enjoyed cooking find that a switch to a vegetarian diet provides an opportunity for them to improve their skills in the kitchen. Joe, a high school music teacher, made the following comment:

> Cooking is more of a challenge. To get the flavors you need to use spices and herbs many people aren't used to using. It's an enjoyable challenge, and you feel really good when you make a meal that tastes really great—like you've got the secret down right.

After learning how to prepare meatless dishes, some people feel that vegetarian cooking is easier and more enjoyable than cooking with flesh. This is because, unlike meat, many vegetarian ingredients require little or no cooking. Others appreciate the fact that vegetarian cuisine is less messy than other styles of cooking; blood and grease are not problems in a vegetarian kitchen.

> Being vegetarian tends to simplify cooking rather than complicate it. I can make a meal of baked or boiled potatoes and yogurt, for example. I make soups and salads often as complete meals for myself. Meatless meals, overall, are faster to prepare than meals that require the cooking of meat.

> I don't like to cook, but I find it easier now. My freezer's not full of meat and I can put something together without cooking. My sink used to have so much grease before, it was splattering all over the wall. Now everything is so nice and clean.

Alternatives to Flesh

Soy products, such as tofu, are an acquired taste for many people, but they make important contributions to the diets of many vegetarians. In fact, a soyfood revolution has occurred in the United States, with literally hundreds of new soy products being developed and released during the last 10 years. These include various brands of soy milk, soy ice cream, soy mayonnaise, and soy hot dogs.

Of all soy foods, tofu in particular is greatly admired. Connie, a chef and caterer, appreciated the versatility of tofu. As she said, "You can do so much with tofu that it's mind boggling. You can scramble it for breakfast, bake it in a quiche, fry it in a wok with vegetables—even make a cheesecake out of it." Although less well known than tofu, tempeh (a cultured soybean product from Indonesia) also has its supporters. As Ava, a vegetarian for 17 years, told us, "I gave up eggs recently and discovered I much prefer thin slices of tempeh browned slowly in a pan with a little soy sauce for breakfast. It's delicious." Peter, another tempeh fan, added, "I enjoy tempeh in sandwiches, in spaghetti sauce, or on its own with a little chili sauce. It's Indonesia's gift to vegetarians."

However, not all vegetarians are in love with soy products. A few unfortunate people have soy allergies. Raw foodists prefer to avoid soy products because they involve cooking. And some people just don't like tofu, no matter how hard they try.

Meat analogues, such as vegetarian bacon, sausage, and hamburger patties, are a debating point among vegetarians. Some find them to be a useful crutch during the early stages of their transition away from flesh. And others continue to enjoy analogues as a permanent part of their diets. In contrast, some vegetarians strongly dislike these products. Many find the flavor and texture of analogues to be disappointing. Typically, these people expect analogues to be exact replicas of meat, but have their expectations disconfirmed with the first mouthful. Shelley, a homemaker and Seventh-Day Adventist, is one of these people:

> In the beginning, some people from the Church said, "Try this. It's imitation meat." I cooked it in a casserole and sat down at the table and thought, "This is going to taste like meat." And it absolutely didn't taste like meat. I thought, "Oh boy. I'm not going to make it."

Other individuals are against the use of meat analogues in principle. Some health vegetarians dislike analogues because they are processed; others are concerned that the large amount of protein they contain is not only unnecessary, but may even cause health problems. Some ethical and aesthetic vegetarians are against analogues because they feel that vegetarians should not eat foods that mimic the texture and flavor of meat. They feel that these products convey the impression that there is something desirable about the eating of flesh and that doing without it is a deprivation.

> Meat analogues are a stepping stone for new vegetarians, which is really good because they have the texture and flavor of meat. The only problem is that a lot of vegetarians stay on that step and don't get off and make the next step. It is healthier to make the next step. Analogues are made of concentrated protein, and our body doesn't need a lot of protein.

> I do not like to hear about meat substitutes, for I think that rather defeats the purpose. The psychological implication is that we'll miss meat, so here is a pacifier of sorts.

Although meat analogues have their detractors, they are useful for several reasons. For one thing, vegetarian patties, sausages, and "hot dogs" allow vegetarians to participate in certain social activities, such as backyard barbecues. Furthermore, the shapes of these products are convenient for cooking and eating. And these foods do not necessarily mimic flesh. As one man asked rhetorically, "Why should meat-eaters have a monopoly on these convenient and familiar food shapes? The original sausage was a banana. Sausage-eaters are imitating vegetarians." Another woman added, "A soybean looks as much like a burger as a cow does." In addition, some of the flavors associated with meat, such as hickory or smoke, are not characteristic of flesh foods and can just as easily be imparted to plant foods. There is no reason why vegetarians cannot enjoy the same flavors, such as hickory-flavored tempeh "bacon," that meat-eaters do.

Although most vegetarians are happy and content with their diets, a few report continuing problems in adjusting to a meatless cuisine. In most cases, these people have only recently become vegetarian and are still missing their favorite meat dishes.

> I think my main complaint about vegetarian food from a taste and texture point of view is that it all seems very much the same. To me, all pastas taste the same, all beans do, more or less, and so do most nut roasts. Although I present things in different ways, I feel that basically I'm always starting with the same ingredients, and the end products are very similar to each other if you close your eyes.

The same problem, of course, occurs among flesh-eaters. Many meats "taste the same" and require sauces or different styles of cooking to impart variations in flavor. Enjoying an interesting and varied diet requires effort and creativity, regardless of what one eats.

Traps for the Unwary

Vegetarians soon learn that many processed foods contain hidden animal ingredients, such as meat stock and lard. For this reason, vegetarians spend a good deal of time standing in supermarket aisles examining the lists of ingredients in products. As one person put it, "I read labels like crazy." Being cautious adds time to shopping, but after a short period of time, people learn which products are "safe." Nevertheless, at one time or another, most vegetarians have been fooled by foods they thought were allowable. Maria, a vegetarian for 12 years, described a common situation:

> It seems that I'm always trying to avoid meat. I mean, almost all processed foods have lard in them. I don't usually buy processed foods, but once in a while at the local supermarket I'll buy crackers or something, and when I get home, there it is: lard. Needless to say I don't buy those brands again.

Although label-reading is a fact of life for vegetarians everywhere, Americans have an advantage in this regard, for the laws regulating the labeling of ingredients in products sold in the United States are more stringent than in most other nations. Consequently, vegetarians in countries such as Australia or England must rely on a certain amount of guesswork.

Reading labels carefully, however, does not guarantee that food is safe. Many vegetarians go for long periods of time before they discover that certain products or ingredients they regularly consume are of animal origin. For example, many vegetarians don't realize that gelatin is made from the skin, tendons, and hooves of animals. Mono- and diglycerides listed in bread or margarine are sometimes of animal origin, and vegetarians need to search for brands that specify plant sources. (One handy tip to remember is that products with the term "Parve" on the label are safe; parve is a Jewish term indicating that the food contains no ingredients of animal origin.)

Without a doubt, the biggest shock for most vegetarians involves cheese. A large number of lacto and lacto-ovo-vegetarians are unaware of the fact that most cheeses contain rennet—an enzyme extracted from the stomach lining of calves. (Rennet is used to coagulate milk into a firm cheese.) Most people feel frustrated and angry upon learning that a food they had always considered to be vegetarian is now off limits. The situation is not totally grim, however, for rennetless cheeses are available in many health food stores and natural groceries, so vegetarians who enjoy grilled cheese sandwiches and pizzas with cheese toppings do not have to go without. Unfortunately, rennetless cheese is usually unavailable in nonvegetarian restaurants, so vegetarians who eat out face a dilemma. Many people we spoke with continue to eat rennet on these occasions. As one person said, "I prefer to eat rennet-free cheese. But I do eat cheese that isn't sometimes. I guess I'm still working on that."

Eating out causes other problems as well. Many vegetarians discover after a period of time that their favorite eating places use animal fat rather than vegetable oil for frying. For example, Richard, a vegetarian for one year, told us that he had eaten french fries at a particular fast-food restaurant for six months before he found out they were cooked in animal fat. When eating out, vegetarians must learn to always ask questions about how food is prepared—even for foods that they assume are safe.

Vegans have a particularly difficult time because milk or eggs are found in so many packaged and baked goods. Extra vigilance is required if they are to be strict about their diets. However, many vegans find that it is necessary to make occasional compromises about what they eat, especially when they are in situations over which they have little control, such as when visiting other people or traveling. The following two comments are from people who are completely vegan at home, but who make small allowances under certain circumstances:

> I would not call myself a true vegan because when I go visiting I take cow's milk in my beverage, and if my host offers a cheese dish—I eat it.

> Sometimes I go out with my friends and get a pizza. I think that's the only time I'll eat cheese. Once in a while I'll have pasta with a cheese sauce at the cafeteria where I work. It's usually just a matter of convenience when a vegan meal is not available.

Some vegans are clear about their reasons for compromising. They feel that the small amount of good done by being 100 percent consistent is not worth the large degree of effort required. Accordingly, they feel that it is better to be flexible than compulsive.

> When I'm eating out I tend not to worry about things like eggs and milk in baked goods. I don't think it's such a big issue. In the end the most important thing is to devote your time and energy to whatever cause you're working on in the most concentrated way possible. If you spend a lot of time worrying if there's an egg in the cake batter, you're losing a lot of time that could be spent in better ways.

> At home we're vegan and have been for twelve years. But being perfectly vegan is such a trial when dining out that I've really loosened up on that. I never eat eggs, but if they've put some yogurt in the dressing or whatever, I just eat it and get on with my life. I can't afford the burden of worrying about what seem like relatively minor details in the face of the whole picture.

Given the fact that animal ingredients appear in so many products, it is virtually impossible to participate in the common culture without "consuming" animals in some sense. For example, the list of goods that contain animal ingredients includes photographic film, cellophane, phonograph records, glue, plastics, paints, ceramics, and automobile tires. People who are serious about vegetarianism need to be strict but realistic about what they can hope to achieve.

Shopping

For vegetarians who are happy to live on simple diets, grocery shopping presents few difficulties; most of the commonly used vegetables, legumes, whole grain products, nuts, and seeds can be purchased in any supermarket. But for vegetarians who enjoy more "exotic" foods, such as soy milk or tempeh, shopping can be problematic. In general, people report fewer problems in large cities than in small towns and rural areas. And in the United States, those on the East and West coasts report fewer problems than do those in the Midwest and the South. However, almost all vegetarians report *some* difficulty. We heard complaints from people living in Pennsylvania, Utah, Virginia,

Colorado, Florida, Canada, and central California that vegetarian food is difficult or even impossible to obtain.

Many vegetarians prefer shopping in natural groceries or health food stores when they are available. However, these establishments are generally more expensive than traditional food stores—an important consideration for people on limited budgets. Jeff described why shopping was often a frustrating experience for him:

> Shopping is a big chore. It's a problem getting supermarkets to carry "health" foods. The local stores have recently started carrying tofu and sprouts, but that's as far as they go. I don't live right in the city, so the health food stores are few and far between, and their mainstay is vitamins anyway. Besides, I cannot afford to buy everything at the health shops—they're too expensive.

Some people who do their shopping at supermarkets occasionally have problems passing the meat counter. Some people complain that the meat department "smells awful." Others find the sight of meat to be unpleasant. As Carl put it:

> If I shop at a supermarket, I avoid the meat counter. It really disgusts me, particularly if people are going on a picnic or something and they have 10 packets of meat. I think, "Oh God, that poor animal."

Food cooperatives, which operate on a nonprofit basis, are an alternative. Some cooperatives have their own premises and full-time salaried employees. Others operate out of someone's garage and involve people contributing a few hours of time on weekends. When organized by vegetarians, cooperatives are capable of providing many products at prices lower than in commercial shops. In small towns where certain vegetarian foods are unavailable, they can make a major contribution to people's daily quality of life. A few individuals in our sample had started their own cooperatives. As one explained:

> We are fortunate in living so close to a whole food warehouse and have set up a cooperative which we organize every couple of months or so. We find it useful to buy in bulk due to the fact that the wholefood shops within a

> thirty mile radius are very expensive and we get snowed in during the winter months.

Organic Food or Commercial?

Most vegetarians, especially those who do their shopping at traditional supermarkets, eat commercially grown produce. However, many individuals are attracted to the idea of eating organically grown food. (Foods grown "organically" use no pesticides or synthetic fertilizers.) Many people feel that organic fruits and vegetables taste better than those grown commercially. Others are concerned about the high levels of pesticide residues sometimes found in commercial produce. Morris, an organic farmer, argued that vegetarians eat more fresh fruit and vegetables than do meat-eaters. For this reason, he felt they should be particularly concerned about pesticide residues. As he said:

> People can eat food laden with chemicals, but because they can't feel it hurting them right at that moment, think there is nothing wrong with it. The more sensitive your body gets, the more you want to keep it healthy. We need to start exposing the dangers of pesticides; then organics would be the trend for popular eating.

Of course, meat-eaters must also contend with this problem, for pesticide residues accumulate in the flesh of cattle, pigs, and chickens. As a general principle, if one is concerned about pesticides, it is safer to eat plant foods, which are low on the food chain, than it is to eat animals, which are high on the food chain.

Not all vegetarians agree that organics are preferable to commercial foods. Some complain about the high cost of organics. Others are concerned about the authenticity of foods labeled "organic." One person pointed out that organic farmers often use "blood and bone" fertilizers made from slaughterhouse by-products—a fact that may disturb some ethical vegetarians. (On the other hand, another person pointed out that pesticide residues from commercial farms are responsible for the deaths of large numbers of wild animals.) And some people who prefer organic produce are simply unable to purchase it in their areas. A solution to these problems was suggested by Maria: "I have a big organic garden, and it's wonderful to be able to go out and get produce that I know is not chemically treated."

Encounters with Meat

By definition, vegetarians eat no meat or fish. However, this does not mean that vegetarians never have occasion to eat flesh. At some point after becoming vegetarian, most people eat meat again, either by accident or design. There are many situations in which accidents occur, for example, at restaurants or potluck dinners. As we pointed out earlier, when most people discover they have eaten meat, their reactions are typically strong and negative.

Nevertheless, a few vegetarians occasionally eat flesh under particular circumstances. Some vegetarians, for the sake of convenience, will order a fish dish if there is no meatless dish on the menu. Others would never order a restaurant dish with meat or fish in it, but eat flesh if it is served to them mistakenly. One person explained her reasoning this way:

> I've eaten meat a couple of times by accident. Occasionally I've gone to a Chinese or a Mexican restaurant and ordered something and thought I'd gotten across to the waiter that I didn't want meat. And maybe a mistake was made or they didn't understand and the dish came with meat in it. When this has happened, I've eaten it because I feel that it isn't going to bring the animal back to life by throwing the meat away. If I don't eat it then the life is definitely going to waste. It's something I've never wished to happen, but when it does, that's how I handle it.

Some vegetarians eat meat occasionally out of politeness. This usually occurs when they are invited to the homes of family members or friends; typically, the host forgets that the person is a vegetarian and serves meat. When faced with this situation, many vegetarians feel awkward and are reluctant to make a fuss, so they eat the food without comment. In these situations, people's reactions to eating meat are mixed, as the following comments illustrate:

> I've eaten meat two times. Both times a long lost friend didn't know I was vegetarian and cooked dinner, and I tried it. And both times I felt really sick and vowed never to do it again. I ate it to be polite mainly, which is stupid, and which I won't do anymore. I thought I was going to die one time. My stomach was cramping terribly and I felt very sick. I just can't digest it anymore.

> The only time I ate meat since I became vegetarian was when I went home to visit my family and my brother—who did not live with my family—didn't remember. He invited me over for dinner and had gone to a lot of trouble and had made filet mignon. And he thought he was offering me something wonderful and I really didn't want to hurt his feelings. So I went ahead and ate it. I was uncomfortable with the idea of what I was eating, but it tasted good, unfortunately. I was hoping it would taste awful.

Although some vegetarians eat meat on the rare occasion, the great majority refuse. As we noted earlier, after being on a fleshless diet for a year or two, most people react to the thought of eating meat with disgust. Nevertheless, accidents do happen, and the occasional mouthful of animal flesh or fat is something vegetarians have to get used to.

Fasting

A few vegetarians, particularly natural hygienists, fast periodically as part of their health program. This is done, it is claimed, to "eliminate toxins from the body." Some people report an enhanced sense of physical—and in some cases spiritual—well-being from this practice. As one woman stated:

> Through natural hygiene, I learned of the benefits of fasting. First I skipped a meal—which I never thought possible. Then I tried one, two, three, six, and seven day fasts on my own. I am convinced of the spiritual as well as the mental and physical benefits of fasting.

Among those vegetarians who occasionally fast, most find it to be a useful practice. However, those who have tried it are not in complete agreement on the merits of fasting. A few gave it up, feeling that it was not worth the effort. And some people just don't like to go hungry. One man told us:

> I was a faster for a while. What I noticed about fasting is that you have all this energy and you're buzzing and you just need a couple of hours sleep. Then I had this experience. I had to go into town because we lived in the mountains. And I looked at myself and I looked terrible. I weighed 110 pounds. My eyes just sparkled and glowed, but the rest of me looked like hell. I said to myself, "Who would want to look like this?" So I quit fasting.

ALCOHOL, TOBACCO, AND OTHER DRUGS

A common view of vegetarians is that they abstain not only from meat, but from alcohol, tobacco, and other drugs. However, this is not always the case. About half of the people we spoke with *never* drink alcohol; most of these are health vegetarians. Another 20 percent drink rarely—about two or three times a year. The rest drink alcohol on a regular social basis, and most of these are ethical vegetarians.

Many people in our sample had been moderate or heavy drinkers who lost the urge to use alcohol after becoming vegetarian. For them, the general improvement in health and well-being that resulted from a vegetarian diet led them to become more sensitive to the debilitating effects of alcohol. Amie, an employee in a natural food store, continued to have the occasional drink, but felt the aftereffects strongly:

> I don't like to drink alcohol anymore as my body has gotten pretty sensitive to toxins and alcohol is one of them. I used to drink to excess when I was in college, but now I don't even like hard liquor. If I drink, I have beer or wine; even then I can feel its effect the next day.

Some give up alcohol, tobacco, and meat simultaneously, as part of a general change to a healthier lifestyle. As Jim, a raw foodist, told us:

> I used to smoke cigarettes, drink beer, and party a lot. I wasn't a degenerate, but I wasn't caring for myself. I was

> abusing myself. When I changed, people said, "You're not going to stick with it. You'll be back here in two months drinking beer." Perhaps their ridicule was extra fuel for the fire. I don't see those people much now; we don't have much in common.

In contrast, other vegetarians continue to drink alcohol with zest. They are not strongly concerned with the health advantages of vegetarianism and feel that alcohol consumption in no way compromises their ethical or social ideals. Greg, for example, enjoyed alcohol regularly:

> I drink beer and wine. I like wine coolers. I feel that it's healthy. It gives me a little zip, and you need a little zip sometimes. I never touch any grain alcohol whatsoever—unless it's mixed, or on social occasions.

Only a small proportion of vegetarians smoke tobacco. Those who do are usually ethical vegetarians for whom health is not a top priority. Some would like to quit smoking, but find that meat is easier to give up than tobacco. A few give up cigarettes but continue to smoke pipes or the occasional cigar.

> I smoked cigarettes when I was younger, but now I've quit. But I do smoke cigars on a social basis. Once or twice a month I'll buy a pack of cigars and pass them out to my friends and I'll have one.

Marijuana smoking is not uncommon in some circles of vegetarians. As one woman told us, "I smoke pot. A lot of vegetarians smoke a lot of pot. Some say it is organically grown from the earth, so how can it be harmful?"

BUT YOU WEAR LEATHER, DON'T YOU?

People often ask vegetarians about their use of leather. Typically, they are searching for an apparent "inconsistency" in the vegetarian's behavior. After all, they ask, "Isn't it hypocritical to refuse to eat animals but to continue to wear their skins?" Of course, the existence of inconsistency depends on one's motives for being vegetarian. The wearing of leather is irrelevant for people who stop eating meat for reasons of personal health; but for ethical vegetarians, the issue of leather is an important one.

Leather is not the only problem. Many novice vegetarians are surprised to discover that numerous nonfood items also contain animal ingredients. For example, most soap contains animal fat, and some shampoos contain animal protein. In addition, cosmetics firms regularly test new substances by placing them in the eyes or on the exposed skin of rabbits. Consequently, many vegetarians who do not wish to harm animals discover that they need to find alternatives, not only to meat, but to a variety of other everyday products as well.

To what extent do vegetarians worry about these issues? Slightly more than one fourth of vegetarians report making an effort to avoid leather and other products containing animal ingredients. These people are mainly ethical vegetarians. However, some health vegetarians also prefer personal care products that contain all natural ingredients, and hence, are not tested on animals. Vegetarians discover that by reading labels, they can usually find alternative products that do not contain animal ingredients. Most women in this group also purchase "cruelty-free" cosmetics, that is, ones that do not involve any animal testing. People who adopt this strict approach put up with a certain amount of inconvenience but feel that it is necessary to be as consistent as possible in living up to their ideals. The following comments of a woman who recently turned vegetarian illustrate this perspective:

> I am working on replacing all my leather products, and my goal is to replace shoes, belts, and bags by the start of next year. I have also stopped buying household products and cosmetics which contain animal products or which are tested on animals in the laboratory. All this change in my consumerism has not been easy. It has been harder, in fact, than changing my diet. It has required time, energy, and commitment to learn about these products and then find them in the market.

Behaving in a manner consistent with one's ethical values can be difficult at the best of times. It is even more difficult when your beliefs put you at odds with the larger culture. Because so many consumer products involve animal ingredients or animal testing, being a consistent ethical vegetarian necessarily involves a degree of vigilance and, occasionally, deprivation. Many women, for example, report being disappointed at having to give up favorite cosmetics or personal care products manufactured by companies that test on animals. Ethical consistency sometimes requires that favorite pastimes or luxury goods be forgone. For example, Rowan, a school teacher, was an avid motorcyclist before he became a vegetarian:

> After turning vegetarian, I started becoming unconsciously uneasy about wearing leather. This surfaced when I faced the dilemma of riding a motorcycle with a piece of cow on my back (a leather jacket). Now my recreation no longer involves motorcycling.

Similarly, Greg, a business consultant, found that his decision to avoid leather clashed with his desire to buy a new car:

> Last week I was looking at a car—a luxury sports car—and it had leather seats. . . . It was the only way I could get it. And it was exactly what I wanted. But the thought of sitting in a car day after day on leather seats . . . I couldn't handle it.

Not all vegetarians strive to maintain ethical consistency. Another group, consisting of slightly less than one out of four vegetarians, would like to minimize their use of animal products but find they usually have to make compromises. Many complain that nonleather alternatives are difficult, or impossible, to obtain. Shoes, in particular, are frequently mentioned in this context. For example, vegetarians who do hard manual labor find that leather boots are a necessity. As one farmer told us, "I can't work out in the fields in Chinese slippers." People in the business world also find it necessary to wear leather shoes on the job; they complain that plastic shoes are uncomfortable, unattractive, not waterproof, and of inferior quality. Karen, for example, told us about her husband's problems as a businessman:

> My husband works in a traditional business environment and hardly anyone knows about our involvement in animal

> rights. He has difficulty buying suits that are not partially wool and enormous difficulty with his feet. He was a runner and developed all sorts of sports medicine problems. So he feels he must wear leather shoes to work. He also feels he has to look normal.

The largest group—representing about one half of vegetarians—continue to use leather and other animal products without concern. Some feel that it would be nice not to rely on animals, but that alternatives to traditional products are too few and far between to make it worth the effort to seek them out. Others simply feel that leather is not an issue; most of these people are health vegetarians.

> I wear leather. I do feel a little guilty about my leather jacket, but I like it too much to give it up.

> I buy shoes made of leather because they're durable. I don't like plastic shoes because they don't breathe. And I don't feel like wearing canvas shoes, especially when I want to dress up.

The question of consistency is a difficult one, and to many vegetarians it is an unresolved issue. Ethical vegetarians may refrain from cosmetics tested on animals and household products that contain animal ingredients, but they may use medical drugs developed through medical research. And, as we noted earlier, animal ingredients can be found in products as diverse as photographic film and car tires. Even something as apparently "safe" as sugar is problematic, for part of the processing of sugar involves filtering it through bone charcoal derived from animals. Making compromises seems to be a fact of life for vegetarians. As one person put it, "If you live in a slaughterhouse, you can't avoid being spattered with blood now and then."

RESTAURANTS

The topic of eating out in restaurants generates a good deal of animated discussion among vegetarians. Restaurant dining is meant to be a pleasurable and relaxing event. But for vegetarians, eating out can be a headache. In fact, the great majority

(86%) report problems, and almost everyone has his or her own restaurant horror story to tell.

By far, the largest complaint is that most restaurants offer few or no meatless dishes. For some reason, the people who plan restaurant menus assume that when people are dining out, they invariably want to eat meat or fish. The fact that even nonvegetarians occasionally prefer a nonflesh meal is rarely acknowledged.

> It is difficult to be vegetarian here in the South. Most restaurants offer few if any choices. Even turnips, black-eyed peas, and butter beans are seasoned with meat.

> Living in a small conservative community has meant that, for all intents and purposes, we had to give up eating in restaurants. There are virtually no vegetarian restaurants, and even the best restaurants have few, if any, meatless dishes.

Some restaurants offer a token vegetarian main course, but these can be less than inspiring. For example, one person told us about the sole vegetarian dish he spotted at the bottom of a dinner menu at a restaurant in a first class hotel. Entitled the "Princess Platter," it consisted of "an assortment of steamed vegetables topped with a poached egg." Not surprisingly, our vegetarian settled for a fruit salad instead.

Vegetarians often find themselves dining with others in restaurants where *every* main course on the menu contains flesh. For the great majority of vegetarians, eating meat or fish is out of the question, so they are forced to either leave (which may be awkward and embarrassing) or improvise something. One possibility is to compose a meal from a few basic side dishes. Many vegetarians, however, get tired of having salads, french fries, and little else to choose from. Another possibility is to attempt to negotiate something with the chef. Sometimes this works out well, but at other times it ends in disappointment.

> There have been meals I've paid a lot for only to still be hungry, such as a fancy French restaurant which served me a heaping plate of green beans. As everyone stopped eating to stare, I made a comment like, "How did they know that's just what I was craving?"

> It's extremely frustrating to go out to dinner anywhere. The average chef seems to think that vegetarian means either the vegetables without the meat or a tray full of cheese and lettuce. I always inform the management beforehand about my dietary needs, but so far I have never been given a nourishing vegetarian meal.

These vegetarian "meals," which reveal little thought or preparation time, are not only boring, but confirm many people's stereotypes that vegetarian food is bland and involves deprivation.

To add insult to injury, vegetarians often pay as much, or sometimes more, for a simple plate of vegetables as do others eating relatively expensive cuts of meat. It is difficult to see any rational reason for this practice, but the "vegetarian meal rip-off" is a common experience. Shelley, a homemaker, offered a good example:

> Once I went to a Greek restaurant and I asked for a vegetarian meal and they didn't know what I was talking about. I said just to bring me the meal without the meat. And I asked them how much the meal would cost and they said $6.95. My husband said, "The meal with the meat costs only $5.95. Why are you charging her more just not to bring the meat?"

Another aspect of the vegetarian meal rip-off is being served portions of food that are smaller than those served to meat-eating diners. Peter, for example, went to a restaurant for lunch with a group of co-workers from a government research agency. Most ordered burgers—the specialty of the house—which were enormous and came with generous helpings of french fried potatoes. In contrast, Peter's spinach quiche—the only meatless dish on the menu—was thinly sliced and came with a piece of lettuce, a slice of tomato, and a strip of carrot on the side. The restaurant appeared to assume that anyone who ordered quiche would have a small appetite. Unfortunately, Peter, like many vegetarians, has a hearty appetite, and the small amount of food he was served didn't even qualify as a snack as far as he was concerned. And, predictably, his lunch was *more* expensive than those of his colleagues.

Another common restaurant problem, referred to earlier, is discovering meat, stock, or animal fat in a meal that is supposed to be vegetarian. Restaurant workers continually forget that "no meat" includes bacon bits, beef and chicken stock, lard, and fish. Many people find that their sensitivity to meat and animal fat increases after they have been vegetarian for several years, and restaurant "mistakes" are quickly noticed:

> My senses of taste and smell are acute. If the muffin tin was greased with bacon fat or the cake batter contains tallow, I know it. If the veggies were cooked on the grill in beef dripping or steamed in chicken broth, it doesn't get by me and I'm filled with revulsion.

Many restaurant workers do not realize that a dish is not vegetarian if it contains animal stock or fat. Because of this problem, many vegetarians routinely question the waiter or waitress about the contents of food, no matter how "vegetarian" the dish sounds on the menu. Asking if foods are fried in vegetable oil or lard is also a good idea. However, some people feel embarrassed doing this. Furthermore, checking first doesn't guarantee that a meal will be meatless, for restaurant workers—even cooks—often don't know exactly what is in the food they serve. Many restaurants buy precooked and packaged dishes that are warmed in microwave ovens before being served to customers. The ingredients in these meals are anyone's guess.

To avoid problems, many individuals only eat in vegetarian restaurants. Of course, this is not a solution for those people who live in areas where vegetarian restaurants are nonexistent.

In contrast to the large number of vegetarians who report that dining in restaurants is disappointing, frustrating, or unnecessarily expensive, a minority—14 percent—claim that eating out continues to be an easy and problem-free part of their lifestyles.

> I don't have any problems with restaurants. There is always something vegetarian or something that can be modified on the menu.

> Eating out has been surprisingly easy and I have been delighted by the number of restaurants, vegetarian and otherwise, who will cater for vegans. And I've noticed, too, that

> many large hotels now include vegetarian fare in their standard menus.

Some people describe experiences in which restaurant workers have gone out of their way to be helpful and accommodating toward them.

> The cafeteria manager where I work asked me one day why I started eating just salads or egg salad sandwiches. I explained that I no longer eat meat, and he began to offer vegetable lasagna, vegetable chop suey and chow mein, and more meatless soups. Although I was flattered, I immediately thought of the number of people who would be healthier for the change.

In summary, views on restaurants vary a good deal. People who are satisfied are thankful that they can generally find something to eat when dining out. Their expectations are not high, and they are happy to get by with a simple meal of salad or vegetables. On the other hand, those who are dissatisfied feel they should, in principle, have the same rights as flesh-eaters to choose from a variety of substantial and tasty meals. For them, another salad or baked potato is not good enough. All in all, it appears that present dining options can be described as tolerable, but with considerable room for improvement. Perhaps the situation would improve if all vegetarians followed the strategies used by Eileen and Janice:

> I speak out in restaurants and tell them it's about time they put a veggie meal on their menu. Whenever I travel for business or pleasure, I support veggie restaurants and tell the hotel where I am staying why I am eating outside of their restaurant.

> I always say audibly that I'm a vegetarian when dining in restaurants. I want the very word to be heard and to become a part of our national vocabulary.

TRAVELING

Closely related to problems in dining out in restaurants are problems in finding vegetarian food when traveling—a situation that can be particularly difficult for vegans. Although a person might know of restaurants in one's home town that provide reasonable vegetarian food, trying to find one in a strange city can be a time-consuming and frustrating task. Situations in foreign countries, where the visitor does not speak the local language, are the most difficult of all. For example, Diane had a job that required frequent travel overseas, and her difficulties as a vegan were considerable:

> My job as an international flight attendant has me eating in restaurants more often than at home. In most cosmopolitan cities I can easily find an ethnic restaurant, but there have been countless experiences where I've had to sift through meals of questionable ingredients to find a few bites of vegetables. I have learned to say "vegetable plate, no eggs, cheese, or meat" in every language. I have a charming way of relaying a message to the chef via the wait person letting him or her know that I'm relying on their creative talent to find something for me and how grateful I will be. Not all the wait people are charmed though, and I can read their expressions of "Why does she even eat out when she has such a restrictive diet?" I agree with them, but I can't pack a separate bag of food for a week, nor do I want to be antisocial with my crew.

In all the international travel experiences we heard, France was mentioned most often as a difficult destination for vegetarians. This is partly a reflection of the fact that French cuisine is heavily oriented toward flesh foods. The following are examples of "French" stories:

> My boyfriend and I went on holidays in Europe for many years, staying first at package type hotels where it was very difficult to get any good food. We lived mainly on melons, lettuce, and French beans, and of course, white bread. It was extremely difficult to get suitable food in France as their ideas on cuisine are so rigid.

> In a Parisian restaurant we pointed to the vegetables on the menu and tried to make the waiter understand that we just wanted the vegetables and not the meat. Our French was very limited. The waiter brought us all nine dishes we had

pointed at—complete with meat. The entire restaurant was looking at our table which was breaking with dishes. This was the first and the last time we went to a restaurant in Paris. After that, we went to the various markets and bought bread, cheese, and vegetables and ate them outdoors.

Having a good grasp of the French language would appear to be a prerequisite for—but not a guarantee of—finding vegetarian food in France. Traveling in English-speaking countries, however, can also be problematic. Jan, an English vegan, described her difficulties in traveling in the United States. American vegetarians who have traveled within their own country can probably sympathize with her comments.

The nearest I've come to starvation was in America. I found it very hard to locate health food shops, and when I did, they were extraordinarily expensive. I spent a week living on corn chips, tea, and Diet Coke, which did me no good at all.

The outlook for tourists, however, is not all bad, and some people describe positive travel experiences. Countries that are particularly congenial to vegetarians include England, Italy, Indonesia, and India. Although few people think of the Soviet Union as an attractive destination for vegetarians, it is possible to eat well there and avoid meat. Jenny, a writer, found that people in her tour group were envious of her Russian vegetarian meals:

I went to the Soviet Union two years ago, thinking I would come close to starvation. And lo and behold, our Intourist guide immediately asked the group if anyone was vegetarian. I think I surprised her with my enthusiastic "Yes!" I was treated like a queen the entire trip. She arranged special meals for me at every stop, and the food, although simple and repetitive, was delicious. Others in the group looked longingly at my plate.

When planning a holiday, it often pays to do some preliminary research, to book ahead, and to make special arrangements with tour operators and airlines. Carla, a nurse, found these steps made her holiday meals problem-free:

> On a recent trip to Nassau, several people noticed my attractive meals which I had prearranged. I enjoyed telling them they contained no meat. Our airline was also very nice and served a delicious vegetarian meal.

Some vegetarians don't realize that it is possible to request a vegetarian meal on most airlines when making reservations or purchasing tickets. The result, however, is variable: Sometimes the meals are excellent, sometimes they are terrible, and sometimes they don't appear at all. Once, for example, Sally, on a trip from the United States to Australia, was served boiled peas, carrots, and a white dinner roll for breakfast, lunch, and dinner. But on another occasion, in Indonesia, she was served an exotic meal with vegetables cooked in half a dozen different styles with rice. Occasionally, as in restaurants, people working for the airlines do not understand the meaning of the word vegetarian and serve inappropriate food.

> I had a vegetarian meal on an airline once. It was chicken chow mein. They must think chicken is a vegetable.

> Even though I had made prior arrangements, I was served a fish. I told the flight attendant that I had ordered a vegetarian meal. She apologized, took the tray away and returned in about 10 minutes. She put the tray in front of me and said, "Here's your vegetarian meal." I looked down. It was the same tray with the same fish on it.

People generally find it is better to tell airline employees exactly what they *can't* eat, rather than say they are vegetarian. Some feel that it is easier to bring a brown bag and forgo the airline meal. But as Carla pointed out, "When you travel you have to make your point politely but firmly, because not providing vegetarian food is discrimination. We have to educate people." However, many feel it is a good idea on long flights to bring food along, just in case the airline "forgets."

COMPANION ANIMALS

Views on companion animals, or pets, are mixed among vegetarians. Many prefer not to have animals at home. Some feel that it is "unnatural" to keep animals in a house or yard. As Benny put it, "I don't have any pets and I don't want any. Animals should be free." John was in agreement: "I wouldn't have a pet myself. I prefer to see animals in their natural state." These people have a "live and let live" attitude toward animals: They like animals but don't feel that humans should interfere in their lives in any way.

In contrast, other vegetarians literally surround themselves with animals. Many feel that the fact that they do not eat flesh allows them to be especially close to their companion animals. As one person put it:

> My animal family now includes three dogs, three pigeons, a goat, a pig, two horses, and several roaming turtles. I love them even more now that I'm a vegetarian. I feel it is a reward for not eating them.

Vegetarians who keep animals often allow them a considerable degree of freedom. To these people, the thought of animals being restrained in cages is unacceptable. Amy, a homemaker, told us about the animals in her family:

> Having pets is a good way to teach love and care of animals to children. We have an aquarium with goldfish and an eccentric parakeet. The parakeet is very tame and will land on your head or shoulder and more or less has the run of the house. He loves to land on the table at breakfast and nibble on bits of cereal or bread crumbs. He is a very affectionate pet.

Having carnivorous companion animals is a topic that generates a good deal of discussion among vegetarians. Some people say they will only keep noncarnivorous animals as pets. One person who feels this way said, "As much as I love and admire cats and dogs, I would never have any because I couldn't stomach feeding them meat." On a more fundamental level, vegetarians who keep carnivorous animals have to deal with an awkward ethical problem: To care for these animals requires that they be fed meat, but meat involves the killing of other animals. This issue is particularly bothersome to animal rights supporters. Should they feed their animals meat? Many do, but feel uneasy about it. One person explained her dilemma:

> I feed my cats meat. I've had a big ethical problem with that. I tried at first to make them something. They have to have some animal protein—milk or eggs. But cat nutrition is very complex, and you can injure the animal if you are not careful. I don't give them pet food that's made from meat by-products, but I give them pet food made from fish by-products, because I believe that if an animal must be killed, a fish is better than a cow. It's not something I feel comfortable with.

Many ethical vegetarians would prefer not to have companion animals. However, they often take in animals from shelters who would otherwise die. Because these animals are carnivorous, the immediate needs of the animals override other concerns. Other people rationalize the feeding of meat to cats and dogs because "it is natural for them to eat meat." As one person put it, "Dogs would be carnivores in nature, so what is wrong with supplying them with what they have in nature?"

Vegetarian pet food is available in some natural food stores. However, many people are reluctant to purchase it because they worry about possible nutritional risks to their animals. Sarah, an animal rights activist and vegan, was cautiously trying out vegetarian dogfood for her animals:

> There is a vegetarian dog food, but I worry a little about it. I guess I'm a little bit brainwashed because I still feed them meat, but gradually I'm changing them over to the vegetarian dog food. As long as I see that they are doing OK.

Many people are surprised to find out that dogs can be raised and maintained as vegetarians. This is because dogs are omnivores—not carnivores—and their natural diets contain plant foods as well as meat. Many of our respondents testified to the fact that dogs do very well on meatless diets. For example,

Stuart said, "I have a vegetarian dog. He is 8 years old. Everyone remarks how young he looks. I just feed him whatever I eat." Will, who lives in a remote area in Australia, also has a vegetarian dog. Sometimes the dog goes into the garden and eats his fill of raw vegetables. Green beans off the vine are his favorites.

Cats, however, require meat in their diets. Robert, a used-car salesman and vegetarian of 17 years, described the mixed results he obtained when trying to feed both cats and dogs as vegetarians:

> We had cats and tried to feed them soybeans. Cats do not eat soybeans. They go out in the woods and catch mice, rats, and birds. We had a couple of dogs. We didn't really want dogs, but they were abandoned, so we adopted them. And dogs will eat soybeans and be quite healthy. But cats—no way. They won't even look at a soybean.

Although dogs can be reared on a meatless diet, cats present an as yet unsolved problem for vegetarian families. (Some people are working on developing a nutritionally balanced vegetarian cat food, but so far the results are unclear.) Nevertheless, vegetarians feel most comfortable when their companion animals are also vegetarians. One of our respondents, in particular, was proud of her completely veganized household. As she stated, "I live with three vegan dogs, three vegan mice, one vegan rabbit, and one vegan husband."

ORGANIZATIONAL INVOLVEMENT

A previous study of vegetarians found that they are more likely than nonvegetarians to be members of clubs or organizations.[1] Many individuals in our sample belong to organizations concerned with the quality of the environment, wildlife preservation, world peace, or the provision of services to the poor. And although a minority in our sample, some individuals belong to groups that specifically promote vegetarianism.

Why do people join vegetarian groups? Some people feel isolated when they first stop eating flesh because they don't know other vegetarians. Local vegetarian groups, when they are available, can serve as an important source of social support. Vegetarian societies are also useful for people who move to new cities because they provide an opportunity to meet and interact with like-minded others. In addition, many vegetarian clubs hold banquets on holidays, providing an alternative to the traditional Thanksgiving turkey or the Easter ham. Finally, vegetarians who are convinced of the rightness of their beliefs can contribute to the spread of vegetarian ideas through participation in an activist organization.

Most large cities in the United States have vegetarian clubs or societies that welcome all types of vegetarians. Some are highly organized, arrange guest speakers, and publish their own newsletters. Others are informal and simply meet occasionally at vegetarian restaurants for a meal. National organizations also exist, such as the North American Vegetarian Society and the American Vegan Society, which stage events and publish newsletters. (Addresses are provided on pages 267–268.) Of course, when local groups are not available, people can start their own. Brenda told us about her experience in forming a vegetarian group:

> We started a local potluck vegetarian group. Since going to it, I've felt great support and have become enthusiastic about vegan cooking. We share recipes and cookbooks. It has been an experience that deepened my commitment to a vegetarian way of life and to the importance of talking to and educating others.

Organizational involvement is important to many ethical vegetarians, particularly those involved in the animal rights movement. Many describe their participation in these groups as a central focus of their lives, because it allows them an opportunity to act on the basis of their beliefs, and because it puts them in touch with others who share this attitude. Many people find that involvement in an organization helps to strengthen their resolve and commitment to their ideals. As one activist put it:

> I spend what time I can with animal rights and vegetarian groups. First for the animals, but also for the social ac-

> tivities and the people. They are the few places I have felt like a member of the family—an extended family of people who accept me because we share the same basic values.

VEGETARIAN COMMUNITIES

A small proportion of individuals live in vegetarian communities. Although it appeals to only a minority of people, communal living offers certain advantages: the sharing of material resources, the pooling of talent, and the provision of companionship. A number of vegetarian communes were founded in the 1960s, and most have since disbanded, but a few have survived into the present.

One example of a successful long-term vegetarian community is that of Gentle World, a group of about 30 ethical and nutritional vegans living in Florida. The community acts as a clearinghouse for vegetarian literature and has published a popular book entitled *The Cookbook for People Who Love Animals*. The residents of Gentle World express strong feelings of camaraderie with their fellow vegans and find a great deal of mutual support in the community. One member of the group told us, "I've met a group of people who for all intents and purposes could be my family. I've never come across a situation where I trust and feel comfortable with so many people."

We also spoke with several people who had lived on The Farm in Tennessee—probably the best known of the vegetarian communes. This group has published several books, including the popular *The Farm Cookbook*. They also produce several soy products, including a dairyless "ice cream," that are sold nationally. Robert described the early days of the community:

> The Farm was vegetarian life on a large scale. When I got there, there were probably about 250 adults. They had all come from San Francisco. Nearly everybody had been turned on to spiritual things through taking psychedelics. It was where all the hippies went. Everyone had long hair. We were a mixture of ex-drug dealers and English and philosophy majors and we didn't have any real idea of how to farm. At first the neighbors were pretty enraged. We

> were like a flying saucer landing in their backyards—like 400 alien hippies. But they saw that we were pretty hard working, and all their kids had left home and moved to the big cities. We were hungry for knowledge and they were delighted. They taught us how to farm.

Although communal life is close and offers a viable lifestyle, it is not suited for everyone. Many people discover that life on an agricultural commune requires a good deal of hard work. In addition, pressures to conform can be strong, and people who have different ideas may be rejected by the group. Questions of privacy also arise, and some individuals feel they are always being observed by others. Not surprisingly, many people "drop out" of rural communal life and drift back to the cities. As Robert said, "I was approximately 30, and in the back of my mind I still wanted to be a millionaire. So I left and moved to San Diego."

Those who choose to live in vegetarian communes represent a very small proportion of contemporary vegetarians. And to a certain extent, these communities are a carryover from the 1960s era of social experimentation. Nevertheless, their emphasis on nonmaterialism and the sharing of resources provides a valuable corrective to the consumerism and individualism that characterize most people's lives.

DEALING WITH INSTITUTIONS

Now and then, vegetarians spend time in institutions, such as hospitals, the military, campus dormitories, and prisons, where their diets bring them into direct conflict with a regimented system. Institutions generally do not make exceptions for people with atypical needs, and this can make life difficult for vegetarians. Patrick, for example, told us about his experiences in the Navy:

> I was in for 2½ years during World War II. Much of that time was on a small minesweeper with 35 people. On those small ships they don't have a regular cook. They have someone who works as a cook but knows little about it. And it was my luck for a while that they had a guy who was a butcher. Naturally he cooked a lot of meat. Another time

> they had someone from the southern states who cooked vegetables with pieces of bacon. So it was difficult for me. There was little that I could eat, and I went hungry much of the time. I lost a lot of weight and I was weak. However, for a time we operated out of New York, and every time we'd go on liberty I'd have a chance to eat. I'd have recuperating periods from starvation.

Hospitals can be intimidating places at the best of times. Many doctors and other health care providers (who are usually not trained in nutrition) have doubts about the soundness of a vegetarian diet. Consequently, they put pressure on vegetarians to eat animal products during their stay. Vegetarians, who may not be feeling well, may be persuaded into going along with their doctors' dietary recommendations. Later, in retrospect, they may regret that they gave in under pressure. For example, Nancy, a vegan, was not allowed to eat her usual diet when she was in the hospital:

> When I was in the hospital last year, the dietician insisted on serving me a heavy lacto-ovo-vegetarian diet which I ate because I needed sustenance. As a result, I felt bloated, constipated, heavy, and generally unwell—not to mention guilty.

Kathy spent time in the hospital after she was injured in an automobile accident. As in Nancy's situation, great pressure was put on her by nurses and doctors to eat meat. But she resisted. The doctors were obviously displeased with her stance, and they wrote in her file that she was a "finicky" eater. She avoided starvation by having friends bring in food. After a period of time, the nurses adjusted to her routine, and they even set aside space in a nearby refrigerator.

Prisons are probably the least flexible of all institutions. Most are overcrowded and operate on limited budgets, making it difficult to cater for individual diets. We spoke with one vegetarian who had spent 1½ years in prison for selling drugs. Not surprisingly, he experienced difficulty in getting decent vegetarian food:

> I was already an established vegetarian when I got to prison. The cooking was awful there. All the vegetables were

> steamed intensely until they turned to mush. If you were blindfolded, you couldn't tell the difference between a carrot and a brussels sprout. If it wasn't for the color of the food, you wouldn't know what it was. However, you could have all the vegetables you wanted. And I invested in protein powder that was sold by the weight lifting club. I would drink a glass of that a day and eat all the produce I could handle, and I seemed to get through there pretty well.

Our respondent also described the reactions of other inmates to his diet. As one might expect, most were not receptive:

> I was the only vegetarian out of 650 men. These guys were felons. I was quite a curiosity and most of these people couldn't relate to it at all. They would ask about it all the time. I'd say that I didn't believe in killing animals, that it was just protein and you could get it in other ways. I'd try to enlighten them, but it fell on pretty deaf ears.

Some prison systems (for example, in Florida) cater for vegetarian inmates. Currently, this is an issue that several vegetarian organizations are working on. Some people might feel that this is "pampering" criminals, but forcing a long-term vegetarian to eat animal flesh might be seen as "cruel and unusual punishment." Besides, because vegetarian food is relatively inexpensive, the provision of meatless meals reduces operating costs. Vegetarian food might even make prisoners more peaceful—an outcome that prison officials would certainly welcome.

EMPLOYMENT

Most vegetarians experience little conflict between their jobs and lifestyles. Sometimes, however, friction occurs. Job-related problems are more common for vegans than for lacto-ovo-vegetarians. Problems are also more common for ethical vegetarians than for health vegetarians.

Sometimes people discover after becoming vegetarians that their diets are in direct conflict with the jobs they have held for years. Some work in restaurants or fast-food outlets that serve meat; others work in clothing stores that sell furs; and still others work in scientific fields that involve animal testing. In many cases, people cannot adjust to the contradiction and leave their jobs to find more appropriate employment. The following woman, for example, went from job to job in a search for a field of work that does not harm animals:

> Through the years I've had to quit jobs on ethical grounds. For example, I was waitressing and felt horrible serving meat, so I quit. I was working retail but the stores sold furs and cosmetics that were tested on animals. Almost every job I've looked into has some sort of negative impact on animals. I'm trying to pass a real estate course right now. If I sell newly developed real estate I will be selling homes to humans on land which used to belong to animals. I can't seem to win.

Similarly, because of their values, some people decline to enter certain fields of employment for which they are qualified. This means that career opportunities are sacrificed. As Jamie stated:

> There are severe limitations on my job opportunities. I am an aerospace engineer and, of course, the Department of Defense is unacceptable now. When one does not even condone the killing of animals, how does one support killing humans?

In a few cases, people are denied jobs because they are vegetarian. The following woman, for example, had her application rejected because of her views about animal experimentation:

> My self-righteousness cost me a job in the Office of Scientific Affairs at the American Psychological Association. I had my membership in the Baltimore Vegetarians on my resume. (It's since been removed.) The interviewer challenged me on it. We descended down the slippery slope of animal rights, and she was a staunch supporter of animal research. Had I been a little more circumspect and a lot less self-righteous, I would have probably gotten the job. However, I doubt if I would have been happy in that environment.

Vegetarianism sometimes causes people to get into trouble with their employers or supervisors. For example, Fran, an elementary school teacher, was reprimanded by her school principal after parents complained about comments she had made about vegetarianism in class. According to her principal, parents were angry because not all sides of the issue had been discussed. As a result of these complaints, the principal warned her never to bring up the topic again. However, Fran's side of the story was different:

> The students had seen me eating tofu, and had been asking me for information on vegetarianism all year. So when the health lesson on the digestive system and nutrition came along, I thought it was the perfect time to respond. The school nurse loaned me a book on nutrition that happened to explain vegetarianism very well. So I decided to read it to my students. A speaker from food services had introduced the topic the day before in her discussion of nutrition and sources of protein other than meat. I devoted only 15 minutes out of a six week unit to the topic. All around my room were cut-outs, mobiles, and pictures of meat. An issue of our reader was devoted entirely to livestock. We also saw a film entitled, "How a hamburger becomes you." I told the children that I do not recommend vegetarianism for children unless their parents are also vegetarian and I told them that being a vegetarian can be difficult. One of the children whose parents complained wasn't in the class that day and so did not even hear what I said. His parents are cattle ranchers.

It appears from Fran's story that as far as some people are concerned, any mention of vegetarianism, regardless of circumstances, is going too far.

Being a vegetarian can also result in problems when food and business are mixed. Business environments tend to be conservative, and being identified as a vegetarian can compromise one's competitive edge in some situations. Of course, one's diet, like one's religion or sexual preferences, is a private matter and should not enter into business considerations. However, people's dietary practices often become obvious because so much business is conducted over meals. Bonnie, a vegan for 10 years, described her approach in this situation:

> Business lunches generally take place at restaurants that have few if any vegetarian entrees. I often have to settle for salads and/or an appetizer or two. And I've made it a rule that my vegetarianism is not a topic open to discussion in the business setting. Too many people are threatened by it. They get on the defensive, and it does not make for the most pleasant exchange. If asked why I'm a vegetarian, my answer is simply "It's a matter of personal preference," and I get off the topic as quickly as possible.

Some vegetarians learn to live with the conflict between their jobs and their beliefs. For example, before she became vegetarian, Trudy worked for a fast-food hamburger chain—an obvious contradiction. However, she was reluctant to leave the company because of the many lifelong benefits it provided. Similarly, Toni told us about her husband's situation:

> My husband and I have been vegetarian for almost one year. However, my husband must also taste recipes which include meat for his restaurant business. He has not eliminated meat choices in his business—he runs a pizza parlor—because he has three partners who are in disagreement on the subject, and because the customer markets in his location would not support such a change.

In a few cases, conflict between people's occupations and beliefs becomes so great that they are fired. Roxanne told us about her experience in radio:

> I was prevented as a news director from covering animal rights stories on our station, so I would sneak them to other media outlets. Sometimes the pressure from other media would force our station to follow suit. Eventually, such activities had a hand in getting me fired.

Although problems are common, the link between diet and employment is not always negative. To the contrary, a surprisingly large number of vegetarians are able to find work that not only is consistent with their beliefs and lifestyles, but allows them to promote vegetarianism in a positive way. Interestingly, vegans are three times more likely than other vegetarians to combine work and diet in this fashion; this probably reflects their relatively high level of commitment.

People with jobs that involve regular contact with the public often use this as an opportunity to speak out about vegetarianism. Maria, for example, is a fashion model who refuses to wear animal furs and participates in cruelty-free fashion shows. In addition to making people aware of alternatives to animal furs, Maria believes that her work helps to dispel certain myths about vegetarians. As she said, "At least people will know we vegetarians aren't skinny and scrawny because of our diet."

To cater for the growing demand for meatless meals, many vegetarians have gone into the restaurant business. Fred, owner of a popular vegetarian restaurant, told us how he got started:

> It all happened about 12 or 13 years ago. At the time I was the owner and operator of a little Mexican fast food restaurant and I got involved in metaphysical training. I did an intensive course that included meditation and yoga. I also became a vegetarian during that time. After that, there was no way I could take pride in my little Mexican fast food restaurant. The first thing I would do in the morning was cook 20 pounds of hamburger for tacos. So I ended up selling the business with the idea of creating a little vegetarian whole food place somewhere.

According to Fred, times were tough in the beginning, but interest in vegetarianism is definitely on the increase. As he said:

> The first few years were difficult. It takes a lot of time to build up a clientele for a specialty restaurant. It seemed all the new information about the effects of what you eat on your health was being swept under the carpet. But now there has been a resurgence of interest. A few years ago we had mainly office workers and students in here for lunch. Now the lunchtime parking lot is filled with Cadillacs and Porsches. Vegetarian eating has moved up market.

Glen, who also owned and operated a vegetarian cafe, agreed that there has been an increase in interest in vegetarian food. As he told us:

> There is more interest in nutrition these days and less emphasis on red meat and fried foods. There are a lot of groups out there plugging healthier diets. And restaurants, all kinds, are gearing toward lighter food, which in a sense cuts into the vegetarian restaurant market. I look at what I'm doing as kind of a service to the community. I don't necessarily like to push vegetarianism, but we have books and will answer questions if people ask. Not all of our clients are vegetarian, but a lot are health-oriented.

Other occupations in which vegetarians are able to combine their beliefs with their work include doctors, nurses, dieticians, artists, writers, farmers, natural food store workers, and food cooperative workers. Some people opt to work full-time in the animal rights movement. One unusual approach is that of Jack and Cherry, who work as "vegetarian consultants." Their work began when Cherry won a recipe contest in a local newspaper—the first vegetarian ever to win the event. After a series of television and radio interviews, a steady stream of people approached them for advice and assistance in becoming vegetarians. One thing led to the next, and they became full-time vegetarian advocates. As they told us:

> We generate enthusiasm for the foodstyle and show people how to prepare good tasting, nutritious meals. For example, when someone is put on a restrictive diet by his or her nutritionist or doctor, we can prove to that person that there is life after meat. We always stress the positive ethical, environmental, and health aspects of vegetarianism. Our weekly half-hour cable TV series "The Vegetarian Kitchen" is designed to introduce viewers to all aspects of vegetarianism and to teach them the basics of vegetarian cooking.

Not everyone can become a professional vegetarian. But the above stories show that it is possible to integrate vegetarian beliefs and practices into many different lines of work.

SUMMARY

The vegetarian lifestyle differs in many ways from the norm. There is no denying the fact that a fleshless diet presents certain difficulties, such as when eating in restaurants, traveling, and dealing with institutions. On the other hand, eliminating flesh from one's diet provides its own rewards, including a discovery of the rich variety of delicious plant foods that are available and a feeling of camaraderie with fellow vegetarians.

The problems described in this chapter largely reflect the fact that vegetarians are a minority group. And like most minority groups, vegetarians are sometimes discriminated against by the majority. However, as vegetarians grow in number, they will make greater demands on the dominant culture. As they gradually modify the society around them, the difficulties associated with the vegetarian lifestyle will undoubtedly decrease in importance.

Chapter 6

Relations with Family, Friends, and Acquaintances

When people first stop eating meat, few realize the full implications of their decision. Most expect that they will have to learn new recipes and acquire tastes for new foods. And most realistically anticipate problems in shopping, eating in restaurants, and traveling. But most fail to appreciate the profound impact becoming vegetarian will have on their relationships with family, friends, and others. Sometimes these changes are welcome and sometimes they are regretted. But regardless of how these changes are felt, almost all vegetarians find that their social worlds are never again quite the same.

DEALING WITH FAMILY

Living as a vegetarian has many implications for one's relations with parents, siblings, and other relatives. Supportive family members, who good-naturedly put up with occasional inconvenience around mealtime, are appreciated by vegetarians. On the other hand, unsupportive family members can make life miserable for both new and long-term vegetarians. The responses of family members typically go through several stages, however, so it is necessary to distinguish initial reactions from later ones.

Initial Reactions

Becoming vegetarian often evokes some sort of response from family members—usually a negative one. In our sample, 66 percent say their parents and other family members were initially opposed to the change, 16 percent claim their families were indifferent, 10 percent say their families were supportive, and 8 percent report mixed reactions—with some family members opposing the change and others favoring it. Family reactions are not related to people's motives for becoming vegetarians; ethical vegetarians are as likely as health vegetarians to meet with family resistance. However, people who adopt strict vegan diets are more likely to report negative reactions from family members than are people who adopt lacto-ovo-vegetarian diets (79% versus 58%, respectively).

Although most relatives have problems dealing with the new vegetarian in their midst, parents, in particular, have a hard time adjusting. Some parents worry about their children's physical (and perhaps mental) health. Other parents are offended because their children no longer partake of certain traditional family foods. Some resent the inconvenience caused. And others simply can't understand—or refuse to understand—the reasons for the change in diet. These problems are exacerbated for young vegetarians living at home, but older vegetarians living away from their parents also catch their share of flak.

The following quotes illustrate some parents' concerns about their sons' and daughters' physical health:

> I met with a lot of opposition from my parents who were raised believing that meat is a necessity. They thought I would be malnourished. I lost some weight after giving up meat, which made them think I was anorexic.
>
> My mother cried. I'm her only son, her only child. She was pretty emotional. She said her image of me was a "cross-legged skeleton meditating somewhere."

Mothers and fathers are especially worried when their children become vegetarians at an early age. Most parents try to force their children to eat meat again; usually they win in the long run, but a few children hold out. The following woman, for example, stopped eating flesh after seeing a farm animal slaughtered while visiting relatives. This led to the existence of a "generation gap" in her family, even though she was only five years old:

> Both my parents were really upset. They thought my diet was lacking in some way and took me to doctors who always said I looked fine. At times I became a real behavior problem. I was very resistant to their attempts to get me to eat meat. I would sit at the table for hours and just refuse. I was a very obstinate child.

Some parents are upset by what they perceive as the "radicalization" of their children. They had wanted nice normal children, but they got vegetarians instead. Some parents respond with a good deal of emotion to their children's unusual behavior. Roberta, a social worker, was unprepared for the strength of her father's reaction:

> My relationship with my father has been very strained. It came to a head last year. He called me "very changed" and said I had became a hippie. He said he used to see me as the logical, goal-oriented one in the family, but not now. I was shocked. He still doesn't accept my lifestyle, although he's calmed down since then. He feels I'm just walking to the beat of a different drummer.

Similarly, Lorna, a university student studying geology, found that vegetarianism led to problems in her relationship with her mother. As she said:

> I got into a few heated arguments with my mother. I did not consciously plan them, but she can be very defensive. For example, I made some Chinese hot and sour soup for myself, and my mother asked me if I had put eggs into it, and I quietly said "No." She became very angry, and soon we were both yelling. She calls me a fanatic.

Some parents are offended and indignant when their children announce they will no longer eat flesh. They see this as tantamount to a rejection of the way in which they raised their children—a rejection that bruises their view of themselves as good parents. For fathers, this impinges on their self-image as responsible providers who work hard to "put meat on the table." Consequently, they resent what they interpret to be ingratitude on the part of their children. Joan, a secretary, was surprised by her father's strong reaction:

> My family reacted very negatively, particularly my father. He is a mellow, pretty agreeable sort of person. And he adored me; I was his princess. But when I first mentioned that I had stopped eating meat, he yelled and screamed and was absolutely furious. Nothing in his life ever made him feel that way. I really touched a nerve. He sees it as an attack on his values and the values of his family. He says, "By God, my parents brought me up to eat meat, drink milk, and get fresh eggs from the farm," and he thinks it is practically holy to eat this way. And for me to imply that this isn't the ideal way to eat makes him absolutely violent.

Some mothers also interpret their children's new diet as a personal rejection. They feel that the care they gave their children by providing nourishing meals for so many years is no longer appreciated. For example, one woman told us how her mother had become very upset when she found out about her daughter's new diet. As she said, "My mother takes personal offense at what I am doing. She loves to cook and feels that I now disapprove of her cooking."

Some parents are annoyed at the inconvenience caused when their children visit and vegetarian meals must be prepared. In particular, they resent the disruption to traditional family events such as Christmas dinner. Parents also become upset when previous family activities, such as hunting and fishing, are rejected by their vegetarian children. As one woman said, "It was a sad day in my father's life when he invited me to join him on a fishing trip and I declined."

Parents in many families are reluctant to understand the change. But some parents reject the idea of vegetarianism so thoroughly that there is little room for discussion, let alone compromise. For example, when Jason stopped eating meat, his father reacted with ridicule and contempt. As Jason told us:

> My Dad used to make fun of my wife and me at meals. There would always be meat for him, and he would hand us the relish tray and say, "Here, this is for you." He was very religious and believed God gave us dominion over animals. My father is a hunter, but even as a little kid I didn't like to hunt. I would comment that I didn't like eating rabbits and squirrels and he would say, "Oh, you're learning all this junk at school; you'll grow up to be a sissy."

In extreme cases, vegetarianism leads to complete breakdowns in the relationships between individuals and their parents. In most of these cases, however, vegetarianism is only one part of a larger set of attitudes and lifestyle choices on which parents and children disagree. Nevertheless, it is often the issue of meat consumption that leads to the final split. As two people put it:

> I see my father infrequently, and if I do, it's usually only for a day or so. He's written me off as such a kook that I don't think that much I could do would faze him.

> My family virtually disowned me years ago on a variety of other issues. Vegetarianism was merely another nail driven into the coffin.

Of course, as we pointed out earlier, not all parents react negatively, and some are enthusiastic about their children's decision to stop eating flesh. When parents react positively, it is often because they are health-conscious and can readily see the value of a low-fat diet centered on plant foods. Occasionally, parents are, or have been, vegetarians themselves. In other cases, parents are active in animal welfare activities and, for this reason, can sympathize with their children's ethical concerns about animals.

Finally, some parents are largely indifferent to their children's decision. Parents who are unconcerned often feel this way because they are used to their children's "eccentricities." Many think that vegetarianism is a passing phase that, if ignored, will go away. As one person said:

> They assumed that it was a passing fad. I was the black sheep of the family. I'd been in prison, I had long hair, a

real nonconformist. They had pretty much burned out by the time I told them I was vegetarian. They said, "We don't care what happens, just enjoy yourself and stay out of jail."

Changes over Time

Most people's parents are less than enthusiastic during the transition to vegetarianism. But over time, many parents who are initially doubtful come to see the benefits of giving up meat, or at least are reassured that it is neither dangerous nor disreputable. Although 66 percent of vegetarians report that their families reacted negatively at the beginning, only 27 percent say their families are still opposed, and 44 percent say their families are now supportive. (In addition, 16% say their families are indifferent and 12% report mixed reactions.)

Although vegans are more likely than lacto-ovo-vegetarians to experience early family difficulties, the two groups are equally likely to report that their families now support their diets. Apparently, families manage to adjust to most vegetarian diets, regardless of how strict they are. And although they may have more doubts about strict diets based entirely on plant foods than about diets that include eggs and dairy products, these doubts are generally put to rest over time. However, ethical vegetarians are less likely than health vegetarians to report that their families are now supportive (32% versus 54%, respectively). Because equal numbers in these two groups report initial family support (about 10%), it appears that families have a relatively hard time coming to grips with vegetarians motivated by ethical concerns about animals. Family members probably find it easier to accept health arguments than ethical arguments for giving up meat.

Given time to adjust, many parents find that occasionally preparing vegetarian food for their children is not as difficult as they had thought. Many realize for the first time that meatless meals can be satisfying and delicious. Some even come to enjoy the challenge, and novelty, of cooking vegetarian food when their children visit. Lynn, a secretary and vegetarian for 10 years, said that her visits home are occasions for her parents to try out new dishes:

> At first my parents thought it was a passing fad I was going through, but in the last five years they have really come to accept it. They even get excited because they can make me something special when I come over for dinner. My father was born in China, and his way is *the* way. He doesn't really listen, but is happy to cook vegetarian dishes when I come over. "Well, whatever," he says, "I just love my daughter."

Other parents come to take pride in their children's attitudes and behavior. For some, having a vegetarian child becomes a mark of distinction. As one woman put it, "At first, my parents were very upset. But now my mother tells people how good it is for you, and how her daughter has been a vegetarian for 20 years."

Many families not only come to see the benefits of vegetarianism, but modify their own diets as well—generally with encouragement and assistance from their vegetarian members. When this occurs, it strengthens the emotional ties between family members. People in vegetarian families often talk about a special bond that unites them, above and beyond the fact that they are related by blood:

> At first, it made me feel a bit estranged because we were on opposite sides of an issue I felt so strongly about. But today, both my sisters have become vegan, as well as one brother-in-law, all my nieces and nephews, and my father. And my mother—the last holdout—is starting to change as well. They have seen me get healthier over the years, and this encouraged them to change. It has brought us all a lot closer together.

Clearly, vegetarianism can lead to major changes in family relationships, with some relationships becoming closer and stronger and others breaking down completely. These opposing trends are illustrated in the following family, where the issue of veganism caused a major schism:

> My relationship with my family was greatly shaken in my early years as a vegan. Those of my family who have adopted veganism are much closer to me than those who haven't. The spectrum of relationships within my family ranges from living with one brother, who shares my diet, to not talking to another for 10 years.

In summary, although few families initially support the change in diet, many come to accept it over time. Positive changes are usually brought about by the vegetarian who, through setting a good example, helps to dispel stereotypes about vegetarians and reveals the diet to be sensible and health-promoting. With encouragement, many families even reduce or eliminate their use of flesh foods. However, for the small proportion of families who do not accept the change, family life becomes more difficult and stressful. Later we discuss some approaches that may be useful in reducing conflict over this issue.

DEALING WITH FRIENDS AND ACQUAINTANCES

We noted earlier that some people have a more difficult time than others during the transition from flesh-eating to vegetarianism. An important factor in this transition is the level of support one gets from friends. Friends who provide sympathy and encouragement facilitate the successful adoption of a vegetarian diet. On the other hand, friends who react with ridicule or disapproval make the change awkward and onerous. For many people, friends are the critical factor that makes an initial experiment with vegetarianism a success or a failure.

Reactions of Friends and Acquaintances

Thirty-four percent of respondents report that when they stopped eating meat, their friends were generally supportive. In fact, some individuals find that a change to vegetarianism is relatively easy because their social circles encourage new lifestyles. As Arlene, a worker in a food cooperative, said, "Most of my friends were natural foods oriented. I didn't have any friends who ate at McDonald's." Others are persuaded to stop eating meat in the first place by their friends. As Fred noted, "The people I associated with were all leaning towards vegetarianism, and, in fact, they were giving me a hard time about this taco restaurant I owned." In the right circles, it can even be an honor to be a vegetarian. As one person said:

> No one has ever criticized or ridiculed me for not eating flesh. Some people in my acquaintance, though not vegetarian themselves, seem in a strange sort of way proud of me. When I've been invited to people's homes, everyone has been glad to know that I am a vegetarian and has provided dishes that I can eat. No one that I know of has ever been offended or put off by this.

On the other hand, many people discover that their friends aren't impressed by a switch to vegetarianism. In our sample, 32 percent of people report that their friends reacted negatively. (Another 16% report mixed reactions—some friends favored the change but others opposed it—and 18% say their friends were mainly indifferent.) The reactions of friends do not vary with people's reasons for adopting a fleshless diet, but vegans are slightly more likely than lacto-ovo-vegetarians to report negative reactions.

Associating with friends who are critical can generate a considerable degree of distress for novice vegetarians. During the first tentative weeks and months, many people feel awkward about their new status and are unsure if their decision is the correct one. They may harbor doubts about the soundness of the diet or whether they will be able to abstain from flesh successfully. Because people are vulnerable during this time, the ridicule of friends can bring the transition to a rapid halt.

When friends are critical, conflict can also result, and it is not uncommon for friendships to break up over the issue of vegetarianism. Sometimes this occurs after a heated argument about animal ethics or religion. More often, vegetarians gradually drift away from those old friends whose values and lifestyles are now seen as fundamentally different.

> I lost all my friends. Then I realized that they weren't my friends anyway. They thought I was crazy and no one wanted to be around me. They would go to eat hamburgers and I wouldn't eat with them. They would drink hard liquor and I wouldn't drink it. It was the best thing to ever happen, to lose those friends.

> I don't have connections with friends back home anymore because there isn't anything we have in common. If we go for dinner they groan and say, "Oh well, looks like we'll have to find something special for the vegetarian." They were brought up on meat and think I'm an oddity.

> My husband and I found ourselves the objects of jokes about our "grazing habits." My husband has been called "wimpy," "dominated by his wife," and "less than a man." Needless to say, we no longer accept dinner invitations from these so-called friends.

Although dealing with old friends can be problematic, the situation is even more difficult when meeting new acquaintances. Sixty-five percent of our respondents report that people generally react negatively when first learning that they are vegetarian. (In addition, 9% report generally positive reactions, 12% report mixed reactions, and 14% say new acquaintances are generally indifferent.) The reactions of acquaintances vary with the type of vegetarian one is. Vegans are more likely to report negative reactions than are lacto-ovo-vegetarians (74% versus 58%, respectively), and ethical vegetarians are more likely than health vegetarians to report negative reactions (74% versus 54%, respectively).

These negative reactions range from amusement or mild criticism to outright hostility. Julie, an English vegan, described the typical reaction she receives:

> I find a lot of people quite hostile when they find out I'm vegan. They tend to dismiss my beliefs without bothering to find out what they are. As soon as they hear that I don't use dairy products, they say that it's "ridiculous" or "stupid."

These frequent negative reactions make some people reluctant to admit they are vegetarians. A few sidestep the issue by saying they don't like meat, are dieting, or have allergies to meat or dairy products.

Although a minority, some people report that others are generally accepting and positive about their diets. These individuals tend to move in relatively open-minded social circles. There is no doubt that some parts of the country are more tolerant of new lifestyles than are others, with reactions tending to be more positive in large cities than in rural areas, and on the East or West Coasts than in the Midwest or South. John, who lived in California, found that most people he met there were interested and supportive of his diet:

> Day-to-day interaction with nonvegetarians is not a problem at all. An astonishing number of them immediately tell me how little red meat they eat, even though I may have said nothing more than "I am a vegetarian." Apparently, lots of people now feel that vegetarianism is a viable and even admirable lifestyle.

Vegetarian Friends

Many people, after they become vegetarians, find that their circles of friends change to a certain extent. As we noted earlier, it is not uncommon to lose old friends after giving up meat. And the desire to be with like-minded others makes people inclined to seek out the company of fellow vegetarians. In fact, the majority of people in our sample say that vegetarianism is a characteristic they look for in new friends. This is consistent with a previous study which found that most lacto-vegetarians and vegans had circles of friends that consisted predominantly of other vegetarians. (Most, however, continued to count meat-eaters as their friends as well.)[1]

Some say that their relationships with vegetarian friends are the strongest they have ever had. Obviously, this reflects the importance of shared values; as a general rule, people tend to be attracted to those who share their attitudes, beliefs, and behaviors. But it also reflects a belief in the goodness of vegetarianism as a way of life, and hence, the goodness of people who follow that way. The following quote illustrates how some individuals feel about their vegetarian friends:

> Many people I had thought were my friends weren't sensitive enough to understand the importance of my decision to stop eating meat, so I lost a lot of friendships. But the new ones that I have made since, because they are based on such strong bonds of kindness, and because I am able to be a much better friend myself, have far surpassed the old friendships. I feel certain they will last forever.

Although having friends who share the same diet is desirable, many people have a difficult time coming into contact with other vegetarians. This is partly because vegetarians are relatively rare, and partly because there is often no established place for them to meet and socialize. In fact, quite a few vegetarians in our sample—some who had been vegetarian for 10 years or longer—had never met another vegetarian. As one of these people who wrote to us stated, "I am unfortunate in that I don't know any other vegetarians to chum up with to enjoy eating. If you have vegetarian friends you have it made."

Persistence is required to find other vegetarians, even in big cities. Vegetarian clubs and organizations, when available, are useful resources. Rhonda, a vegetarian for six years, described how she eventually tracked down some vegetarian friends with the assistance of several organizations:

> Socially, I felt alone for a long time. Nearly a year ago, I began to reach out. Through the Baltimore Vegetarians and the North American Vegetarian Society, I obtained the name of a contact person in Ohio. I wrote to him and he provided me with a local contact. From that came my involvement with a local animal rights organization and pleasant relationships with the vegetarians in this group.

As Rhonda's case illustrates, ethical vegetarians often make contact with others by joining animal rights organizations. Glenda described her happiness at finally finding a group of people who share her views:

> Shortly after getting divorced, I found a small animal rights group, many of whose members were vegetarian. It was the most wonderful feeling to find other people who share my beliefs about animals after 10 years of isolation as a vegetarian.

Another common pattern is for isolated vegetarians to move to communities or areas that are relatively accepting of new lifestyles. Many of the vegetarians we interviewed had moved to California because they felt it would be easier to meet other vegetarians there. For example, Amy moved to California from the Midwest. Shortly after arriving, she met other people who shared her interest in natural foods. As she said, "The West Coast is such an easy place to live. It is definitely a plus to live in a health place where you are not seen as a kook."

Problems in Socializing

Vegetarians tend to be sociable people. A previous study of vegetarians found that they socialize and entertain, on average, more than do nonvegetarians.[2] Like most people, vegetarians enjoy socializing with others who share their attitudes. However, other vegetarians are relatively scarce and hard to find—particularly in some parts of the country. So, in spite of the potential for disagreement, the great majority of vegetarians continue to interact socially with meat-eaters. This usually does not result in major problems; nevertheless, some vegetarians have mixed feelings about doing this. They feel that although they are more or less accepted by their meat-eating friends, a degree of tension is always present in the background. This tension is felt by both parties, as the following quote from Julia, a homemaker, illustrates:

> As I began to feel more comfortable with being vegetarian, I realized that other people feel awkward around me. Almost everyone has respected my lifestyle, but it still seems to make them feel uneasy. It's sometimes hard for me not to feel defensive.

A variety of problems are encountered by vegetarians who socialize with meat-eaters. Some feel annoyed when jokes or insensitive comments are made about their diets:

> Everyone we know who is not a vegetarian thinks it is odd. They sort of snicker behind their hands, and when they are through laughing about it, they usually act concerned

> about our 5-year-old son, implying that we are depriving him.

Although most vegetarians agree that there is more to a relationship than what you eat, some express disappointment at seeing their friends continue to eat flesh. They believe that eliminating meat is an obviously worthwhile goal and are frustrated or hurt when friends choose to ignore their example. The realization that they are different from their friends causes some to feel isolated or lonely—even when in the company of others:

> At times it is difficult being vegetarian and dealing with others who do not accept my beliefs. I try not to alienate or antagonize my friends. And I will not intentionally give up friends of many years because they do not share my beliefs. But at times it is lonely feeling different and being called weird. And it hurts me that people whom I respect do not "see the light," so to speak.

> I am by nature a sociable type and sometimes I feel very isolated and distant from people I like because of my attitudes towards animals. And it hurts me constantly—the conflict inside caused by people I like going hunting and having barbecues. I mostly keep relating to them in as many ways as I can.

Almost all vegetarians have had experiences with meat-eaters who want to debate them. A typical strategy used by these people is to challenge vegetarians to justify apparent inconsistencies in their behavior. For example, they may ask vegetarians why they wear leather or wool, or how they can justify the killing of plants or insects. Their goal is to reveal the vegetarian as a hypocrite. According to vegetarians, however, these argumentative meat-eaters are rarely interested in a sincere exchange of views. For one thing, they tend not to be good listeners. And their antivegetarian arguments often are simplistic. As one respondent put it, she was tired of hearing about "the cabbage that screamed." Not surprisingly, ethical vegetarians are more likely than others to wind up in heated debates with antivegetarians. The comments below illustrate some of the ways in which people deal with these situations:

> Since becoming older, I do not encounter the baiters so much. They are the ones who ask you how you know a carrot doesn't feel pain or how you can eat in a restaurant that serves meat. When I get this, I explain that I do the best I can and that it is impossible to avoid all aspects of animal cruelty.
>
> When people find out you're vegetarian they want to know if you take antibiotics or kill cockroaches. They're looking for any sort of inconsistency. What they don't realize is that the existence of inconsistency in a person has no bearing on the validity of the ethical argument. It is a primitive way of dealing with ethics.

The issue of consistency bedevils vegetarians. Ethical vegetarians try not to harm animals, but sometimes, directly or indirectly, their actions have negative consequences for animals. This is simply unavoidable in a culture that depends as much on the use of animals as ours does. Similarly, health vegetarians may occasionally eat junk food or drink alcohol. However, the existence of a single inconsistency doesn't make a person a hypocrite; everyone occasionally acts in ways that are not in full accordance with his or her values. Yet, to the continual annoyance of most vegetarians, people pounce on the slightest evidence of inconsistency in a vegetarian's lifestyle as "proof" of their insincerity. As Philip asked, "No one is perfect, so why should vegetarians be subjected to such thorough cross-examination?"

Sometimes, of course, people are genuinely interested in learning about the vegetarian diet or lifestyle. Nevertheless, the barrage of questions is often irritating. Diane, a flight attendant and vegan for four years, described what it was like to be the center of attention constantly:

> My main peeves are those tiresome questions of "What do you eat?", "Where do you get your protein and calcium?", "Do you take vitamins?", and, worst of all, "Do you eat chicken and fish?" I answer the questions if they are sincerely asked, but I back off from those who try to challenge me. I've even had room service waiters hang around after delivering a vegan meal wanting information. Being

> vegan in public is apparently admitting that you are public domain and anyone can ask you personal questions, put you on the spot, make fun of you, worry that you won't get enough to eat, or talk to you while you are eating.

Recent converts to vegetarianism are often enthusiastic about discussing their diets. But the topic is more interesting to the meat-eater than to the long-term vegetarian. Some vegetarians eventually get tired of discussing the topic whenever they eat with others.

> When I try to order at a restaurant, it invariably comes up. The first question is usually, "What do you eat?" Then comes, "What ever made you decide to do such a thing?" Most people don't think twice about demanding an explanation from me. I end up spending most of the dinner explaining and/or defending vegetarianism. I don't mind the explaining, but sometimes I'd just like to eat in peace.

Vegetarians often comment that they don't mind discussing their diets or their reasons for abstaining from meat if people are genuinely interested in changing their behavior. But little good appears to come from most of these conversations. As Frieda said, "I get frustrated and feel let down continually explaining my philosophy to others and finding that no one has ever bothered to make any changes."

Dining with Nonvegetarians

Eating with meat-eating friends and family, especially at their homes, can be awkward. Some vegetarians feel that it is an imposition to have to state a condition (that is, no meat) before accepting a dinner invitation. This feeling is especially common among new vegetarians who haven't gotten used to making special requests for food. But vegetarians eventually discover that it is best to tell people what they will and won't eat in order to avoid mixups. As many learn through experience, a little embarrassment initially can help to avoid greater embarrassment when a meal is served.

How do others react? Arlene nicely summarized the range of reactions that vegetarians encounter:

> When we dine with friends and family we have encountered three approaches to dealing with our different eating habits. One, they go the "full hog" and prepare a delightful, delicious, totally veggie meal. Two, they cook as they normally would, so you have to do with the side dishes and salad. Three, they assume that if you have no choice you will eat the meat.

Most vegetarians say that their friends and family make an effort to accommodate them when dining. This is greatly appreciated. The following woman, for example, reports that members of her family try hard to ensure that she is always well fed:

> I have a sister-in-law who truly goes out of her way to prepare an extra vegetable or a special casserole for family parties. Other family members put themselves out and study vegan recipes, even making sure that there is vegan margarine instead of butter. I feel very touched. It is wonderful to be accepted unconditionally.

But not all friends and family are adaptable. A small group of people find that friends or family members stop inviting them to dinner after they become vegetarian. Some individuals don't want to invite vegetarians to dinner because they claim they don't know what to cook. Others seem to feel that if vegetarians are going to make life difficult for everyone, then they don't deserve an invitation. The following woman, for example, found her sister to be uncooperative:

> My sister stopped inviting me to dinner. She said, "I don't know what to feed a vegetarian." She is always telling me about how her other relatives come over for barbecues and how good it is. Naturally, I'm not invited. Her idea of a good meal is a big steak only cooked a couple of minutes so there is still blood in it. Her husband has had radical heart surgery—five or six by-passes. Now they have been told to have more meatless meals.

A small group of vegetarians do not accept invitations to meals if they know that meat will be served—even if vegetarian food is available. For some, the sight and smell of flesh foods fills them with disgust. As one person said, "Watching people chew on bones is intolerable." Others avoid social occasions when meat is served to "protest" what they perceive to be immoral behavior. As one person put it:

> I do not accept dinner invitations with family members, especially holiday dinners where a dead bird will occupy the center of the table. I feel no remorse or apology for this. My family doesn't like it, but I don't particularly like to have violence on the table.

A common problem that occurs when eating at others' homes is dealing with "hidden" ingredients (a situation often encountered in restaurants as well). Many meat-eaters do not realize that most vegetarians are strict about not eating *any* product derived from animal flesh, and sometimes "just a little bit of stock" or some other ingredient finds its way into meals. This can result in embarrassing situations in which vegetarians have to decline dishes, even though they appear to be meatless. Daphne told us about an incident that occurred to her: "One not so funny experience was when my sister-in-law strained the meat out of the spaghetti sauce for my husband and me. We think she missed the point." Similarly, Peter told us about an elaborate vegetarian meal that a friend had prepared. All was going well until dessert, when the host served a dish that contained gelatin. Although gelatin is made from animal skin and tendons, Peter ate it graciously. As he said, "She didn't realize what gelatin is made from, and to have refused to eat it would have embarrassed both of us. I just tried not to think about it."

Some vegetarians are disturbed to find that family members or friends try to force meat on them or deliberately sabotage their diets:

> My mother was so irritated with my not wanting to eat meat that one day she asked me to close my eyes and open my mouth. She said she had something special for me. I closed my eyes and ended up with a meatball in my mouth.

Family pressure tends to be strongest at holidays. And of all holidays, Thanksgiving is mentioned most often as being difficult. For most vegetarians, the "Thanksgiving dinner problem" is an annual event:

> My family thinks I'm crazy. Every Thanksgiving they say, "Oh, come on. Aren't you going to try a little bit? You don't know what you're missing." I say, "Yes, I do. That is why I'm not eating it."

A similar problem was reported by Alisa, age nine and a vegetarian from birth, who didn't see eye-to-eye with her meat-eating stepmother:

> My stepmother seems to be dying for me to eat meat. On Thanksgiving day she said to me, "I hope some day that you will be able to be a true American and eat turkey for Thanksgiving." Just as she finished she picked up a turkey part and showed it to me as if I couldn't see it myself. I guess true Americans don't have any concern for animals.

A few lucky vegetarians have sympathetic families who are happy to prepare meatless holiday meals—even at Thanksgiving. The following person, for example, described how his mother's Thanksgiving day meals have become well-known events:

> My parents, who are not vegetarian, graciously serve me veggie meals. In fact, my mother's Thanksgiving dinners have gained a reputation among my friends who beg to be invited. On account of one son's persuasion, every year one less turkey's neck meets the butcher's knife.

Problems are less serious when vegetarians invite meat-eating family and friends to dine at their own homes; under these circumstances, vegetarians have complete control over what gets served. However, at times, dinner guests can be unappreciative and even downright rude. Some refuse to try dishes that include unusual ingredients, such as tofu or whole grain pasta. Others denigrate fleshless meals by claiming that they do not "feel full" after eating.

> We expend a lot of energy preparing elaborate vegetarian meals when we have dinner parties. Once, one of our friends said, "Oh, that's nice, but I never really think a meal is a meal unless it's got meat in it." We stopped inviting him over for dinner after that.
>
> I have a problem with people who refuse to try my spinach lasagna. And I once had guests who went out for hamburgers as soon as they left my place.

The issue of whether or not a vegetarian should pay for a meat dish when taking friends or family out to dinner at restaurants comes up occasionally. Some vegetarians feel that it is dictatorial to set limits on what others can and can't eat at restaurants. Consequently, they are happy to purchase meat for friends and family if that is what they wish. On the other hand, other vegetarians feel that their friends should respect their dietary practices, particularly if they spring from ethical or religious beliefs, and they prefer that nonvegetarians not order and eat meat. Nevertheless, these people sometimes find that friends and family members place them in awkward situations by ordering flesh foods. In these situations, many vegetarians simply pay the bill and say nothing, even though they are disappointed. A few, however, refuse to pay for meat under any circumstances. As Rosalyn put it, "If I'm treating friends, I explain to them that they wouldn't get flesh at my home dinner table, so I can't in good conscience buy it in a restaurant."

Why Some Meat-Eaters Are So Obnoxious

Why do so many meat-eaters react with curiosity, derision, or hostility when they encounter a vegetarian? Many of our respondents had explanations for the meat-eater's constant fascination with vegetarianism. Many, such as Anna, believe that meat-eaters are defensive because they feel that their own lifestyles and values are being implicitly devalued. As she pointed out, "People get very offended if you appear to criticize their diets because their diets are part of who they are—another representation of themselves, like their clothes or hairstyle." Others suggest that some meat-eaters are touchy because, in the backs of their minds, they feel guilty about eating animals. Valerie, a vegan for 12 years, put it this way:

> I can see that some people feel uncomfortable—and even guilty—around me because my reason for being vegan is a reverence for life. If you're a health vegan, people can say, "I don't eat much red meat anymore." But if you are an ethical vegan, they would have to say, "I don't do much killing." It sounds different.

A few suggest that meat-eaters don't listen too closely to pro-vegetarian arguments because they don't want to be influenced. After all, if meat-eaters find they agree with the reasons for abstaining from meat, they might have to change their own behavior. This means they would have to give up flesh foods, which they enjoy.

> Most of my friends respected what I was doing but didn't want to become vegetarian themselves. They were interested but didn't want to hear the gory details. If I wanted to do it, fine, but eating meat is pleasurable and they wanted to be able to continue doing it without feeling guilty.

And of course meat-eaters, like most people, are averse to admitting that they are wrong. The ethical arguments for vegetarianism, in particular, deal with fundamental values. Many people do not wish to consider the possibility that the killing of animals for food might be morally wrong, because this would require rethinking many issues. Consequently, they may engage in denial to avoid having to grapple with difficult questions.

> People have to face themselves when they see you doing something different, and some find it a little difficult. Perhaps it is their egos. They might have to agree that you were right all along, in spite of the fact that they ridiculed you along the way. And I have a feeling that people who make a big deal over vegetarianism have a problem with killing. They don't want to face it because it is a threat to the way they think. No one wants to admit they have been wrong in their values.

As the number of vegetarians increases, and as public understanding of the issues underlying vegetarianism grows, vegetarians should have an easier time socially. To a certain extent, this has already happened. Vegetarianism has become more acceptable in recent years due to the fact that the general public has become increasingly health-conscious. Many people are presently aware of the benefits of good nutrition, avoiding cigarettes, and getting regular exercise. Although concern about one's physical well-being used to earn one the label of "health nut," today it is simply viewed as common sense. As a result, vegetarians have come to feel less rejection and hostility from the larger community than they did in the past. As one long-term vegetarian said, "I've found that over the years, people see that I am very healthy and athletic, and they generally have heard something good about vegetarianism, so there is a lot more acceptance now."

Living Arrangements

Although most single vegetarians prefer to live with other vegetarians, a large proportion in our sample live with meat-eaters. For many, it is simply impossible to find compatible vegetarians with whom they can share accommodations. (We discuss relations between vegetarians and meat-eating spouses in Chapter 7.) The ideal strategy for dealing with meat-eating housemates is to convert them into vegetarians. Sometimes this strategy is successful; several respondents told us that they converted anywhere from one to an entire household of people to a fleshless diet.

Most vegetarians, however, have to learn to live with the cooking of meat. Not surprisingly, this often results in problems. The most common complaints vegetarians have about living with meat-eaters include: the nauseating smell of cooking meat, the sickening sight of raw meat, the extra cost meat adds to the food bill, the cleaning of greasy kitchenware, and the impossibility of sharing meals. One woman was concerned that having meat in the house could be a health hazard, particularly if prepared carelessly:

> I do a certain amount of cooking for my roommate, which involves preparing meat—chicken or fish, usually. This is not pleasant to me, but there are several reasons I do it. One is that he is totally unconcerned about washing his hands, counters, or utensils when handling meat. On Thanksgiving Day, I observed him handling the raw turkey, rinsing his hands in cold water with no soap, and wiping his hands on his pants. It did not bother him to touch doorknobs and light switches and possibly spread germs all over the house. If I prepare foods, the risk to both of us is minimized.

In spite of occasional problems, many vegetarians claim that living with meat-eaters is not difficult. As Susan said, "I have always lived with nonvegetarians and it doesn't bother me. Most of the people I live with don't eat a lot of meat." Benny had a similar point of view: "No, there aren't any problems. If anything, I think my roommates have gained through living with me. Sure, I don't like the smell of meat cooking or reaching for a greasy sponge, but that's just little stuff." The experiences of most people show that despite some fundamental differences, peaceful coexistence is possible between meat-eaters and vegetarians living in the same household.

The Extended Visit

Staying with nonvegetarian family and friends can be problematic because, as a guest, one generally doesn't have much control over what goes on in the kitchen. If the hosts happen to be gourmet vegetarian cooks, then the visit will undoubtedly be smooth. However, preparing fleshless meals can be a strain for meat-eating hosts who are not familiar with vegetarian cooking—and this includes most of them. This means that, in most cases, other arrangements must be made. As one woman complained:

> Visits to my meat-consuming family present a problem. I have to either cook separately, make do with the nonmeat side dishes, or go to the local all-you-can-eat salad bar and spend money I would rather not.

Having family or friends to stay can also be problematic. Although most meat-eaters can survive the occasional vegetarian meal, many feel deprived if they are forced to go without meat for too long. Sometimes the disparity between the eating habits of vegetarians and their house guests can make meals awkward and stressful, leaving both parties feeling dissatisfied.

> I enjoy having our family to stay but being the only vegetarian I am sometimes nervous about serving the meal. I won't cook any meat and have had to put up with unadventurous relatives not willing to try new things.

> When my parents visited, my mother was happy to go to a vegetarian restaurant, but my father would just make huge scenes. He would speak very loudly about how he wanted a steak and ask, "Where can we go to get some real food?"

How do vegetarians handle nonvegetarian house guests? There are a number of strategies. The most direct one is simply to forbid meat in the house. People who adopt this rule feel they have a basic right to have their views complied with in their own homes.

> I would absolutely not let anyone cook meat in my house. I would say, "No, I'm sorry you can't. If you want to go home, cook it, eat it, and then come back, that's fine."

> In the past, guests coming to visit would be requested to cook their animals in separate pots. Now, since I own my own home, no meats are cooked here at all. If people want to eat meat they can go out and eat it.

This strategy has the advantage of being clear and simple, and it is unlikely to lead to misunderstandings. However, it can also estrange friends and family members.

Others allow meat in their homes, provided that their guests do the cooking. In some cases, luncheon meat is seen as a reasonable compromise because, compared with cooked meat, it doesn't produce offensive smells or leave cooking utensils greasy. Bill found a different, but convenient, solution to this problem. As he said, "My wife's brother comes to stay once in a while and he loves bacon in the morning, but bacon is particularly smelly. So we give him a hot plate and make him cook it outside."

A few vegetarians don't mind cooking meat for their visitors. These people tend to be health rather than ethical vegetarians. As they see it, a host's duty is to make his or her guests as comfortable as possible. For them, catering for the needs of family and friends is more important than a commitment to a meatless household.

Although the extended visit can be awkward, vegetarians generally find that a good house guest is one who causes as little disruption and inconvenience as possible, regardless of who is visiting whom. When visiting, and when being visited, vegetarians who explicitly state their needs, including what they will and will not eat, help to keep potentially embarrassing situations from arising.

STEREOTYPES OF VEGETARIANS

Stereotypes about vegetarians, both positive and negative, are common in our culture. Some probably contain an element of truth; but like most stereotypes, they are exaggerations. The following is a selection of some of the stereotypes people in our sample had encountered:

> Some people see vegetarians as other-worldly, kind of frail, in a state of bliss, floaty, and in general, not connected with reality.
>
> Say "No" to meat and most people think you are crazy, a wimp, in need of motherly advice, or a threat to their lifestyle.
>
> People who have unusual diets are generally perceived as cranks, health faddists, or just plain un-American.
>
> Most people think vegetarians are pale and anemic. I heard a comedian one time and he said, "Are there any vegetarians out there tonight? Oh, it's OK. I know you're too weak to clap."

> People think that all vegetarians are health nuts, but that is not true. I know some vegetarians who like nothing better than Fritos and cookies.

Stereotypes fill a number of social and psychological functions. Because most stereotypes are negative, they allow individuals to dismiss entire groups of people and not take them seriously. For example, individuals who believe that vegetarians are all "health nuts" are unlikely to consider the positive health implications of a low-fat fleshless diet. And people who consider vegetarians to be "sentimental animal lovers" are unlikely to listen carefully to the ethical arguments for not slaughtering and eating animals. As such, stereotypes allow people to protect their own beliefs about meat and animals by distancing themselves from vegetarians and the values they represent.

Of course, most vegetarians do not fit the stereotypes that are common in our culture. Some vegetarians say that others are often surprised because they don't look or act like the "typical" vegetarian.

> I'm told I don't look like a vegetarian. But just because I'm more comfortable in an evening gown than jeans doesn't mean I have no moral character. I would like to know what a vegetarian looks like anyway.

> Sometimes people have heard stories about me: no cigarettes, no alcohol, no coffee, tea, or chocolate, no meat, no eggs, no honey, mostly raw food, and so on. People expect me to be some kind of Gandhi. When they meet me, they are shocked. I happen to be a 200-pound, happy, healthy, aggressive, male animal.

Some meat-eaters find the idea of not eating meat so outrageous and foreign to their way of thinking that they literally don't know what to make of it. Consequently, they react with shock or amusement when meeting their first vegetarian. For example, Sal told us the following story:

> I went back to see my grandmother in Oklahoma and to accommodate my diet we decided to go to Wyatts cafeteria, where you pick and choose what you want. I asked the person behind the counter what things were vegetarian

> and she just cracked up. In fact, she went in and brought out all the other employees and she said, "Look. Do you want to see a vegetarian?" and they were all laughing. It was amazing. I didn't take it personally. I thought it was funny that they thought it was funny. But still, it was a bit freakish.

Although stereotypes about vegetarians are widespread, attitudes toward vegetarianism are changing. Many long-term vegetarians comment that people's views are less stereotyped now than in the past. Robert, a salesman and vegetarian for 15 years, commented:

> A lot of people think vegetarians are skinny and spacey. But more people are starting to see vegetarianism as healthy. I think the "airhead" stereotype is disappearing because the vegetarians who were airheads have gone. All the people who were on unhealthy fad diets are also gone. Perhaps they've passed away.

In most cases, vegetarians are relatively normal people living a sensible and viable lifestyle. As Diana said, "Vegetarians are just normal people with above normal vision—a vision that is readily acquired, not inherent." With enough interaction between vegetarians and nonvegetarians, these stereotypes will eventually disappear and "ordinary" people will be persuaded to take the diet more seriously.

THE MISSIONARY VEGETARIAN

Before concluding our discussion of social relationships, we consider one further question: To what extent do vegetarians attempt to convert others to their way of life? To explore this issue, we asked people about their attempts to persuade or convert meat-eaters. As it turns out, most vegetarians do feel some obligation to inform others about the benefits of vegetarianism. Eighty-seven percent of people in our sample say that they have tried to influence others to give up or eat less meat. As two people put it:

> We have a moral duty to inform people gently, not to forcibly push it, but at least to let them know there is an alternative, and to inform them of the detrimental aspects of eating meat.

> I am learning more all the time and feel it is part of my duty as a vegetarian to know as much as I can, not so much for my own health but to be knowledgeable and helpful when others ask me questions, as they frequently do.

Vegetarians differ, however, in their beliefs about the best way of accomplishing this goal. Forty-two percent are active and direct in their attempts to persuade others. These people are more likely to be ethical than health vegetarians (51% versus 17%, respectively).

> I am a fairly militant vegetarian. I find it difficult to keep my mouth shut when the opportunity to speak out comes up. I have alienated some people. I regret this because I would rather keep the lines of communication open. But that's just me. I feel so strongly about this that sometimes I can't control my mouth.

Just as some nonvegetarians are argumentative, so too are some vegetarians. They welcome a good debate and adopt a confrontational style when the issue of meat consumption is raised.

> I don't think people's feelings should be spared when it comes to eating animals. The animals' feelings were never spared. People should not be shielded from what they are eating.

> The really persistent ones usually get a description of a slaughterhouse guaranteed to shut them up. The problem with that is that then no one feels like eating.

Other vegetarians, however, feel that the direct, forceful approach makes people defensive and, for this reason, is not very effective. Instead, they prefer to use diplomacy. Many started off being argumentative in their early days, but as they gained more experience, they became more subtle in their attempts to persuade others of the benefits of a meatless diet.

> Like most recent converts, such as ex-smokers and dieters, I went through my self-righteous period, calling meat "dead animals" and drawing people into arguments about ethics, health, and the like. During that time I read quite a few books, so I had plenty of ammunition. Over time I got over my self-righteousness. I came to understand the difference between discussion and proselytizing.

Directly trying to persuade people not to eat meat is often ineffective. Consequently, many vegetarians (45%) prefer to set an example, rather than directly confront others with arguments. They say that setting an example leads to sincere questions from meat-eaters, and this creates an opportunity for an amicable and productive exchange of views.

> I have noticed that my personal behavior is a much more effective way to let nonvegetarians become more aware of how meaningful vegetarianism is, rather than preaching to them or admonishing them for their attitudes and behavior. I try to set a positive example.

> I work hard at not making others feel uncomfortable in their own lifestyles. I've found that setting a strict and consistent example breeds intelligent questions and dialogue that plants necessary seeds of change.

Some people find they gain the respect of meat-eaters by showing tolerance and by not trying to force their views on them. And because they are respected, they are in a good position to exert real influence on their friends' beliefs.

A minority of 13 percent say they do not feel that it is their role to try and change other people's minds. For these people, vegetarianism is a private matter that they prefer not to talk about. As one person put it, "I just let people go on their own way." These people are more likely to be health than ethical vegetarians (26% versus 6%, respectively).

How successful are vegetarians at converting others? Most vegetarians can point to at least one person whose behavior they have influenced in some way, and some people are strikingly successful at introducing new members to the ranks of vegetarianism. The fact that one might be a small force for social change is a good reason for not shutting meat-eaters out of one's circle of friends. Helping others to adopt a healthier diet is a rewarding experience for most people. When this happens, it helps to make all the social difficulties vegetarians encounter easier to bear.

Chapter 7

Vegetarianism and Intimate Relationships

Given the strength and pervasiveness of the personal changes that accompany the transition to vegetarianism, it is not surprising that becoming a vegetarian has major consequences for people's intimate relationships. For single vegetarians, dating meat-eaters can pose problems, and sometimes vegetarians find themselves in romantic relationships with people who share neither their diets nor their beliefs. Relations between spouses are invariably affected if one partner becomes vegetarian and the other does not. Tension between partners is the usual outcome and can lead, in extreme situations, to the destruction of the relationship. And raising children as vegetarians is complicated for both parents and children.

In all of these situations, vegetarianism poses challenges and potential difficulties. However, it also provides opportunities for further growth in close relationships. As we will see, vegetarianism can both divide people and bring them together.

VEGETARIAN DATING DILEMMAS

Our study reveals that most single vegetarians prefer to date other vegetarians. However, because vegetarians are relatively rare in the population, single vegetarians generally have problems finding eligible partners. This problem is particularly acute for women because they strongly outnumber male vegetarians. Slightly more than half the respondents in our sample (51%) are single, and of these, three fourths complained of the difficulty involved in locating suitable dating partners. The two women below, one a health vegetarian and the other an ethical vegetarian, expressed their frustration in trying to find the right man:

> There are so few vegetarians that I've never met any who have shared other interests in my life. They mostly seem to be female too. So, when considering "marriage partners," it is difficult to find someone who has similar eating habits and values.

> I would have a difficult time getting along with a man who is not involved in animal ethics. It is not so much whether he eats meat or not, but whether he is potentially convertible. It is difficult to find men with that frame of mind.

However, men also have a hard time finding vegetarian women, and in our sample, they are as likely as women to complain about dating problems. Donald, who lives in a rural area, told us:

> I am a single father with three sons. I am sharing land with two other vegan males. I think it's peculiar that [among] three vegan males we have not met one vegan female who was single. That has been the biggest disadvantage, I'd say, of the lifestyle that we've chosen.

Dating problems are equally likely to be reported by ethical and health vegetarians. However, the level of difficulty experienced increases with the strictness of one's diet. Finding suitable dating partners is difficult enough for lacto-ovo-vegetarians, but the problems are even more challenging for vegans, natural hygienists, and fruitarians. John, a 33 year old raw foodist, voiced his complaint:

> Dating someone seriously is a problem. There are not many people who have the same interests that I do, who eat mainly raw fruits and vegetables—and organic on top of it. Also, I'm not into material things and spend a lot of time outdoors. My life is simple and that seems to me to be a drawback as far as dating is concerned.

Most single vegetarians are acutely aware of the limited number of available dating partners. A 40-year-old vegetarian divorcée provided the following pessimistic, but realistic, assessment of the vegetarian dating game: "It is hard enough finding eligible men. If you think you can find a vegetarian on top of it all, all I can say is good luck."

Vegetarians Only?

As a result of these difficulties, certain standards develop among vegetarian singles as to the "acceptability" of potential partners. These standards vary a good deal from person to person; with the question of who one dates, as with the question of what one eats, some vegetarians are stricter than others.

Nearly half of the singles in our sample (49%) steadfastly refuse to date meat-eaters—no matter how lousy their social lives are. Some of these people are not only revolted by meat-eating, but by meat-eaters as well. Many mention that they can't stand the thought of kissing someone who has recently eaten meat.

> It is difficult for me to have a boyfriend who isn't vegetarian. You don't want to kiss someone with greasy pork fat on his mouth.

> I couldn't be attracted to someone who includes meat in his digestion. It is repulsive to me.

> The thought of crawling into bed with a woman—even an attractive woman—who eats meat is repellent.

Others comment that they only date vegetarians because they do not want to become romantically involved with people who are on different ideological or spiritual wavelengths. As we noted earlier, vegetarianism is more than a diet; it is a fundamental aspect of people's lifestyles and identities. For this reason, many individuals feel that it would be difficult or impossible to feel close to someone who does not share this trait. For example, one woman said, "I can't imagine being seriously or sexually involved with someone who is not a vegetarian. It is fundamental to all I hold true." Along similar lines, another woman commented, "I find carnivores unappealing. I can't give my heart to them, so why give my body?"

Making Compromises

To avoid a nonexistent love life, slightly more than half of single vegetarians (51%) say they date meat-eaters. However, about half of these compromisers (27% of all single vegetarians) add qualifications. Some say they go out with meat-eaters, but do not allow themselves to get seriously involved. For these people, meat-eaters are people to do things with until the "right" vegetarian comes along. Andy, age 31, put it bluntly: "Meat-eaters are OK for one night stands. But that's all." Marilyn, age 25, described it this way:

> It depends on how serious I want to be with someone. I would go out with a meat-eater for a short term relationship—as long as I didn't have to watch him eating meat. Longer than a couple of months, then it would become a major problem. Eventually, I would want someone who is vegetarian.

Other individuals date meat-eaters—but only if they hold similiar values, are sympathetic to vegetarianism, and are good candidates for conversion. These people say that as the relationship develops, they would expect their partners to adopt a vegetarian lifestyle. If their partners failed to change, however, the relationship could not continue. As Brenda, age 27, said:

> Unlike some of my single friends, I don't find it difficult to be single and vegetarian. I would not refuse to date someone who ate meat, but he would at least have to be sympathetic. If he wasn't, I doubt that I would be dating him in the first place, because a clash of values would be readily apparent at the first meeting. I would hope that over time he would learn from me, adopt a vegan lifestyle, and internalize the underlying philosophy, because I could never allow meat into my home, and my philosophy is a very important part of who I am.

Vivian, a vegan, found herself in a relationship with a man who claimed to be sympathetic to vegetarianism. However, she sensed that he was not sincere. Because of the importance of the issue, she decided to end the relationship rather than take a chance. As she explained:

> I was once involved with a man who kept saying that he was madly in love with me, but he wasn't a vegetarian. He said that if we got married he might eat meat out, but would not have it in the house. I didn't buy it. I've seen too many marriages in which this is a sore point. It's such a deep choice in a person's life—not the same as not eating sugar or not drinking coffee.

Finally, 24 percent of singles say that diet doesn't enter into their decisions about dating partners. For them, vegetarianism is desirable, but by no means a necessity, in forming a relationship. Interestingly, women are more likely than men to feel this way. This probably reflects the fact that there are fewer male than female vegetarians in the dating pool; hence, women cannot afford to be as selective as men in their choice of dating partners. People who feel this way are as likely to be health vegetarians as they are to be ethical vegetarians. However, health vegetarians do expect their meat-eating dates to be health-conscious; meat-eaters who smoke cigarettes, drink alcohol, and get their exercise mainly by changing television channels are not welcome. As Henry, a 36-year-old advertising executive, said:

> It doesn't matter to me that much if a woman eats a little meat now and then, but I wouldn't want to go out with someone who isn't concerned about her health. I'm physically active and like to be with women who share my interests. Sitting on a bar stool all night isn't my idea of a good time. To me, smoking cigarettes is just as bad as eating meat.

Problems in Dating Meat-Eaters

Many single vegetarians find that, like it or not, dating nonvegetarians is a necessity. Not unexpectedly, this can result in problems. For one thing, vegetarians frequently complain about having to watch their dates eat meat. On a deeper level, it is on these occasions that disputes over values are most likely to arise. For many couples, a "romantic dinner" serves as a reminder of a major lifestyle difference between them and foreshadows future problems in the relationship.

Some dates are surprisingly insensitive to the strength of many vegetarians' feelings about eating meat. For example, a female animal rights supporter had the following experience:

> I had a date take me to a restaurant called "The Butcher Shop." It was a place he liked to go and he knew I was vegetarian. I said, "I don't care if this place has a salad bar, I'm not going in there." He got really cranky about it, but I didn't care. It was really stupid of him in the first place.

Amy, a health-oriented vegetarian, was feeling dissatisfied with her love life. She had tried on several occasions to get the men in her life to stop eating flesh, but with little effect. As she said, "I've felt frustrated with some men I've dated who wouldn't take the time to consider changing their diet—not for me but for their own health."

The obstinacy of many men in refusing to give up a "macho" diet of meat and potatoes is a sore point among many vegetarian women. As Joan, a secretary and ethical vegetarian, put it:

> Most of the men I have dated have not been vegetarian and are not willing to go to health food restaurants. They want to have their meat and potatoes or they're not happy. I find most men very resistant to even talking about it.

One should not get the impression from the above comments that it is always vegetarians who reject meat-eaters; the reverse also happens. Sometimes vegetarians are rejected by potential dating partners because their meatless diets are seen as being too restrictive. The following quote is from Julie, a beautician and vegetarian for 10 years:

> I've had people walk away from me—especially real macho, egotistical men. The first thing that comes to their mind is, "I won't get a steak dinner out of her" or "I can't take her for a steak dinner," and they are turned off. I've felt bad about it at times.

All in all, the prospects for vegetarian singles are limited. Vegetarian partners are few and far between, and the ones who are available are often not compatible for other reasons. Consequently, most singles compromise. Some are happy to "get their kicks" by dating meat-eaters, but save their hearts for ideal vegetarian partners. Others are willing to go out with potential "pre-vegetarians," but reject meat-and-potatoes types. Finally, some are willing to give anyone a try, regardless of diet or attitudes. The extent to which one is willing to compromise appears to reflect the priority of vegetarianism in one's own life.

LIVING TOGETHER: SPOUSES AND DE FACTO PARTNERS

Most single vegetarians say they would prefer a vegetarian spouse if they were to marry. However, for many vegetarians, things don't work out this way. About half (49%) of the respondents in our sample are married or in de facto relationships. Of the women in this group, slightly more than half have spouses who eat meat. The pattern is quite different for vegetarian men, with only about 20 percent having meat-eating partners. This difference reflects the fact that more women than men are vegetarian. It also reflects the fact that in relationships, men are less likely than women to change to accommodate their partners.

Vegetarian Couples

In a few instances, both members of a couple are vegetarian before they meet. Claudia and Paul, for example, had each been raised as vegetarians from birth. Interestingly, they met at a vegetarian disco in London which Paul was operating. For couples such as these, maintaining their lifestyles is relatively easy and there are few problems.

In other cases, one person is a meat-eater at the time the relationship is formed and the other is a vegetarian, but the meat-eater later changes. The conversion of a lover or a spouse is a happy moment in a vegetarian's life:

> My wife was raised in a Hindu household in Fiji. But when she went off to school in India she began eating animals. She reverted back to vegetarianism in order to marry me, and she vowed to remain vegetarian. Over the last two years she has become inspired by her newfound reasons for vegetarianism and accompanies me to nearly all of our animal rights protests. I am very proud of her.

Sometimes both partners are meat-eaters when they meet or marry and later discover vegetarianism together. In a few cases, both are lacto-ovo-vegetarian at the time they partner and later become vegan together. Making the change with a partner, as opposed to doing it alone, tends to make the transition relatively easy and enjoyable. In addition, these couples generally find that it brings them closer together and strengthens their relationship.

> My boyfriend and I gave up meat together. Since the day that we cooked one last meat meal, we have greatly enjoyed learning about vegetarianism together. The change was very easy because we could support each other and there was no conflict. We're both strongly committed to vegetarianism as a way of life and this helps cement our relationship.

In most cases, couples make the transition together because it is something they both want. In other cases, one partner persuades—or coerces—the other into trying a fleshless diet. Despite a few sparks in the beginning, these arrangements sometimes work out well in the long run.

> My wife had a bunch of meat in the freezer and one day I came home and threw it all out. She said, "Why did you do that?" and I said, "Because we're going to be vegetarian." She said, "Oh yeah? I didn't know that." Then she really started getting into it, and she cooked a few dishes. Pretty soon she could cook really well. She converted completely.

> When my wife came home and said she was becoming vegetarian my immediate reaction was, "Oh nooo." But I got used to it. She changed before I did, but I quickly saw the light.

Mixed Couples

A large proportion of vegetarians—41 percent in our sample—live with spouses who do not share their diets or their convictions. The typical case is one in which a woman decides to become vegetarian sometime after she has begun to live with her spouse. In many cases, the new vegetarian feels let down and frustrated when her partner refuses to share her enthusiasm. In addition, meat-eaters are often skeptical about their spouses' beliefs or diets, and many are openly hostile. This, as one would expect, usually leads to conflict. The following woman, for example, found that becoming a vegetarian led to a deterioration in the quality of her relationship with her husband; she must have had a very strong commitment to have withstood the barrage of manipulative tactics and ridicule to which he subjected her:

> At the beginning my husband was so angry I couldn't even explain my reasons. He still thinks my stand against meat-eating is stupid and says it will not make one bit of difference to the number of animals slaughtered. He tells everyone that he eats twice as much meat to make up for what I am not eating. When we travel he gets angry because I am eating pasta primavera instead of our old pattern of ordering "chateaubriand for two." He says he gets no joy from eating out anymore because I cannot share in what he is enjoying. Our friends would also say (always in front of my husband), "We would love to have you for dinner, but now that you're vegetarian I wouldn't know what to cook." These comments always added more fuel to my husband's argument that my decision to become vegetarian was an inconvenience to everyone. I would feel anger at these uncreative people making an issue out of something that is absolutely no problem to me. No matter how much I tell people that I love salads, rice and vegetables, they would make an issue over it. I wish I had some vegetarian friends. My husband is so opposed it makes it very hard for me.

Although the above story is distressing, it is not atypical; altogether, we noted problems in 85 percent of mixed marriages. These situations are particularly troubling for women who continue to prepare and cook meat for their husbands—either because they feel it is their duty or because they are pressured by their husbands. Imagine the daily distress of one woman who said, "I find it difficult to cook meat for my husband. Touching it gives me the creeps. After all, it is the flesh of a murdered nonhuman animal."

To make matters even more difficult, living with a meat-eater sometimes generates problems, not only within the relationship, but among wider social circles as well. Ethical vegetarians, in particular, sometimes feel that they are looked down on by other vegetarians because they are "fraternizing with the enemy." Some vegetarians are embarrassed by the fact that their partners continue to eat meat. However, others are also irritated by what they perceive as unnecessary intrusions from others into their private lives. The following woman felt that she had had a hard enough time coping with her flesh-eating husband without having to put up with the criticisms of others:

> I have lived with him for the last ten years and he has lived with me through the process of my giving up meat. It has not influenced him, unfortunately, but if I make a bean burrito he will eat it. I get angry if others make some offhand remarks about my living with a meat-eater. I would rather it were different but it is my private life and nobody's business.

Many husbands are unswayed by their wives' arguments for vegetarianism. Consequently, for some women, it literally comes down to a choice between divorce and tolerating their husband's "addiction" to meat. Most women realize, realistically, that their chances of finding a new vegetarian spouse are slim. And of course, their husbands may have other redeeming virtues. So most couples eventually reach some sort of compromise. Many of these compromises work reasonably well, although a degree of tension often persists below the surface.

Compromises usually involve a decrease in the amount of meat eaten at home. In our sample, 59 percent of husbands had cut down their consumption of meat in response to their wives' urgings. The most common arrangement is for husbands to eat vegetarian meals at home but to order meat when dining at restaurants. In other cases, husbands agree not to eat meat in the presence of their wives.

> My husband, whom I regard as one of the best and most moral people in the world, is not a vegetarian. I will not reproduce our quarrels. They were serious. The outcome of them is that in our house and whenever he is with me, my husband is vegetarian. Period. My latest pronouncement is that anyone who eats meat must be willing to slaughter or at least witness the slaughter. I said this to my husband who disagrees with me that vegetarianism is a necessary outgrowth of caring about cruelty and animals, and he did not respond. Perhaps he is thinking about it.

Husbands vary in how well they accept this compromise arrangement. Some enter into it grudgingly. Because their wives refuse to buy or prepare meat, and because their wives are usually in charge of the shopping and cooking, these men become de facto semivegetarians—whether they like it or not. Other husbands continue to eat meat as often as they can, but accept their wives' vegetarianism without complaint—a situation with which most wives are satisfied. In other cases, meat-eating husbands are strongly supportive, basically accept their wives arguments, and voluntarily cut down their own consumption of meat. Sharon, a vegetarian for one year, found her husband was very positive about the change:

> Luckily for me, my husband has been supportive of my diet change and views. Although he continues to eat meat, it is less. He says he hopes to be a vegetarian someday and is in full support of raising our children as vegetarians.

In some instances, husbands prepare separate meals for themselves at home when they feel like eating flesh foods; this typically occurs in "shared" marriages in which household chores are equally divided between spouses, and husbands are used to doing a good deal of cooking. These egalitarian marriages, because of their flexibility, are better able to adjust when the wife stops eating meat than are traditional marriages in which the wife is expected to do all the cooking. As Margaret said, "When my husband wants to eat meat, he cooks it himself. But most of the time he is happy to eat vegetarian food. He has even learned to prepare it himself."

Occasionally, odd problems develop in mixed couples, as the following story illustrates:

> My husband eats meat. We had established a relationship before I had completely given up meat and I promised him I wouldn't try too hard to change his lifestyle. After 8 years he eats a little less meat but mainly for reasons of weight loss. We do have one problem though which is annoying to me. Because I eat no meat, I find the smell of it on another person's breath to be horrible. He can smell up an entire room, simply by breathing. Sometimes at night I have to open up all the windows and turn up the fan. I make him gargle constantly. His friends joke, "Sleeping alone tonight?" when he orders a burger. It is mainly beef that I find really offensive.

Some vegetarians believe that giving up flesh is a personal decision that should not be made because of social pressure. Accordingly, they do not feel that it is their role to force their spouses to change. The following woman, for example, didn't want her husband to be a vegetarian "imposter" merely to please her:

> My husband doesn't agree with me that it is cruel and still eats meat at restaurants. But he is slowly changing, although I try not to force him to change. I would prefer that [he do it because] he thought it was cruel rather than because I want him to.

When Relationships Fail

In a small number of cases, compromise is not possible, and differences in values related to vegetarianism lead to the complete collapse of the relationship. Of course, division over the issue of vegetarianism usually indicates deeper problems in the relationship and often reflects the fact that the couple has been growing apart for some time. Nevertheless, it is sometimes an argument over meat-eating that initiates the breakdown. For the two women below, the issue of vegetarianism was an "irreconcilable difference":

> I was married to a meat-eater but am now divorced. Should I marry again he would have to be vegetarian. There were certain problems involved with our differences of opinion. Mostly, I didn't want my children to eat meat and he did. I didn't even want it in my house and I didn't like to cook it.

> My husband was a meat-eater. He was aware of my beliefs, but we never discussed it much. In the beginning, I would cook meat for him, but after about one year I grew to the point of refusing to buy, touch, or cook it. We couldn't agree on whether to raise our future children as vegetarians or meat-eaters. This, along with other problems, convinced us to divorce after two years of marriage.

Divorce is inevitably an unpleasant experience, but for some women, getting rid of meat-eating husbands is also a relief. After the divorce, these women feel they are finally free to live as they wish, without having to put up with the objections and ridicule of their spouses. The daily hassle of cooking two separate meals is seen by some as a symbol of the emotional and philosophical distance between partners. As one woman said, "The most difficult thing about being vegetarian was cooking a vegetarian meal for me and a meat meal for him. When I dumped my husband, the cooking got easier."

Two people in our sample—one woman and one man—found that being vegetarian was used against them in divorce proceedings and was a factor in their losing custody of their children. It is difficult to comprehend how a judge could use vegetarianism as a criterion for refusing custody to a parent, considering the medical evidence showing that meatless diets are nutritionally sound and healthy. Nevertheless, in cases such as these, poorly informed judges may fear that vegetarian parents will neglect their children's health. They may also erroneously believe that vegetarians are members of bizarre religious cults and fear that vegetarian parents will instill "deviant" values in their children. The following story is a good example of how being slightly unusual can result in discrimination from those who enforce the status quo:

> When we married, she knew I was mainly a vegetarian, but then I used to eat fish. She kept eating meat and I kept progressing towards a pure vegetarian diet. I would teach the children what sugar does to them, what's in their meat and what salt and preservatives do to them. She knew she had to divorce me or the children would say, "Why don't you follow Dad?" I didn't get awarded the kids in court because the judge thought I was weird. She divorced me and a lot of the problem was over food. I was represented in court by my wife's psychiatrist as being paranoid because I didn't trust the food system or the water system. I'm a very social person and they said I was paranoid. I thought it was a compliment.

For the following woman, vegetarianism became a troubling and critical issue in the disintegration of her family:

> I have been married twice, becoming vegetarian and then vegan in my first marriage. This I thought was a joint decision until the divorce when my husband made it clear that he had only gone along with me [because] I seemed to him so dominant. This came as a great shock to me, and although I fought hard for my two sons in court, he gained custody. He turned back to junk food and meat-eating, which was very hard for me to come to terms with as I had tried to teach them the wisdom of veganism and healthy eating.

Living with a meat-eating spouse is a fact of life for many vegetarians, and most adjust to it. But even after adjustments are made, it remains a source of tension in most relationships. For these people, there doesn't appear to be any ideal solution, short of converting the spouse—which may be impossible—or leaving the relationship—which may not be desirable. Of course, few marriages are perfect, and many spouses gain benefits from each other and enjoy mutual activities in spite of frequent disagreements and conflict. As in dating relationships, the degree to which people are comfortable with compromise reflects the centrality of vegetarian values in their own lives.

MEN, WOMEN, AND VEGETARIANISM

The fact that the majority of vegetarians are women suggests that men and women have different attitudes toward eating meat. The finding that many husbands continue to eat flesh despite their spouses' strong objections also indicates a major difference between the sexes. The general reluctance of men to embrace, or even tolerate, vegetarianism complicates the intimate relationships of vegetarian women, be they single or married. What makes men so attached to eating meat?

The Socialization of Men and Women

Differences in the upbringing of boys and girls may account for the general reluctance of men to consider vegetarianism. For one thing, boys are not encouraged to show emotions such as sympathy, compassion, and gentleness; instead, they are expected to be tough. In contrast, these values are instilled in young girls to prepare them for future roles as nurturers and caregivers. In adulthood, many men find it difficult to empathize with others and express tender feelings. Furthermore, many fear being labeled "soft" or "tenderhearted" because these are seen as female qualities. Consequently, for many men, appeals to compassion for animals are rejected as mere sentimentality.

In addition, encouraging boys to hunt and fish teaches them that it is acceptable to hurt and kill animals. Girls, on the other hand, are taught that it is not nice to pull the legs off bugs and that they should be kind to animals. For these reasons, most men grow up to believe that nature is meant to be dominated and exploited for their own benefit. Consequently, males are less likely than females to develop a reverance for life or to value peaceful coexistence with nature. For men, becoming a vegetarian requires renouncing their domination over animals—an attitude which many are reluctant to adopt.

Another factor is the misperception among men that meat-eating makes them strong and virile—an image that has been exploited successfully by the meat industry. However, as we pointed out earlier, it is complex carbohydrates, not protein, that supply energy for hard work. In fact, a large number of middle-aged meat-eating men are overweight, suffer from hypertension, and are on the road to coronary bypass operations—hardly a macho he-man image. Also, it is not uncommon for meat-eating men with cholesterol-laden arteries to have heart attacks as a result of exertion during lovemaking, suggesting that meat-eating is anything but an aphrodisiac.

Women, more than men, are taught the need for self-control. After all, girls are frequently told that it is not "ladylike" to behave in certain ways, whereas boys are more often allowed to run wild. This may make it easier for women than men to exert the self-restraint necessary to abstain from meat. In addition, because women have less status and power than men, it may be easier for them to adopt a socially unpopular stance; after all, they have less to lose than men do.

Husbands, Wives, and Vegetarianism

All in all, men are more resistant to vegetarian arguments than are women. Nevertheless, the reluctance of husbands of vegetarian wives to modify their consumption of meat is curious. Becoming a vegetarian, or at least a semivegetarian, is not, when all is said and done, that difficult. Furthermore, many meat-eating men live with staunch animal rights supporters who think that eating meat is immoral and cruel. Why are these men so unresponsive to the good models provided by their wives?

The balance of power between women and men in our society is certainly a factor. Women's opinions are seen by many as carrying less weight than those of men; consequently, some men may dismiss their wives' deeply held beliefs as being trivial. A related issue is that of dominance within marital relationships. If becoming vegetarian is the wife's idea, some men may feel threatened by what appears to be a show of independence and oppose it in order to maintain control. Some vegetarian women feel that the issue of control has some bearing on their husbands' unwillingness to become vegetarian. As one woman said, "My husband likes most of the meals I cook but he still eats meat when we go out. I think he is embarrassed in case people think I have control over him."

The following woman's story illustrates how people exert pressure on married men to maintain control:

> I met an old friend from high school and he and I shared a lot of interests. Peace for animals was one he agreed with after many night-long conversations. He became vegetarian for himself, not to please me. I was impressed. We decided to get married about three months later. Soon after our decision to marry I found out I was pregnant. His family thought I had pushed him into everything: vegetarianism, animal rights, marriage, and parenthood. They give him too little credit for having a mind of his own. He doesn't agree.

In the above example, people might have objected less if the situation were reversed and the wife had followed her husband's ideas.

The reluctance of men to stop eating meat means that many wives and girlfriends fail to become vegetarians, even though they would like to. The following woman told us that her father was the main obstacle blocking her mother's desire to become a vegetarian:

> My father knows that if he wants to go to a fancy restaurant, I am going to embarrass him by asking for a special platter. My mother wants to eat a lot less meat. She loves vegetables and would like to order what I order, but Dad is so domineering. He says, "Oh, come on now, that's her thing. You get the roast beef." She would have the vegetables if he didn't say anything.

Ironically, nearly all the major books describing vegetarianism have been written by men. The vegetarian movement today, in this sense, is similar to other movements in history, such as the antislavery movement: Men write about it and take much of the glory, but it is mainly women who act and make up the rank and file of the movement.

RAISING VEGETARIAN CHILDREN

Many people—including vegetarians—feel uneasy about the idea of raising children on meatless diets. The very thought causes a variety of perplexing questions to come to mind: Can children get the proper nutrients necessary for growth without meat or other animal products? Will children eat vegetarian food without complaint? Will children be able to understand and accept their parents' reasons for being vegetarian? What will happen in social situations, such as at children's parties? Will children be rejected by their peers? And what about those interfering in-laws? We spoke to and received letters from 66 vegetarian parents, and their experiences allow us to provide some answers to these questions.

Children's Health

Dieticians and nutritionists say that children can be raised in good health as vegetarians; as with adults, all the essential nutrients necessary for children can be obtained from well-balanced diets that do not include meat.[1] However, children, because they are growing, have greater nutritional needs than do adults. Consequently, some experts recommend that, to be on the safe side, vegetarian children be given certain dietary supplements, including iron, zinc, calcium, and riboflavin. In addition, vegan parents should supplement their children's diets with Vitamins D and B-12.[2] Vegan parents should also ensure that their children get adequate calories, as plant foods are generally lower in calories than are foods of animal origin. Parents who wish to raise their children as vegetarians should do some preliminary reading or consult a dietician. Vegetarian parents, like all parents, should feed their children with care.

What do the parents in our sample say? Of all parents raising their children as vegetarians, none report that their children ever suffered from any diet-related health problem. In fact, 70 percent of parents claim that their children's health is above average—better than the health of their children's agemates who eat meat. Of course, this could be a "proud parent" effect, but the absence of any negative accounts is noteworthy. Some parents comment that, because they are raising their children as vegetarians in a skeptical world, they made sure they knew a good deal about child nutrition before they started. Others say they are particularly careful to make sure their children always eat health-promoting foods. Agatha, who raised her children to adulthood on a vegan diet, is a good example:

> Gone were caffeinated beverages, sugary and fatty junk foods, the incessant eating between meals, the heavy and complicated dishes covered with gravies, sauces and butter. We instituted regular exercise and family outings in nature. Our two children grew up without broken bones, carious teeth, illnesses, disciplinary problems or stunted growth. Our son grew up to be slightly over six feet tall on this diet, just like his father who grew up on meat, milk, and potatoes.

The following is a selection of three parents' comments about the health implications of raising children as vegetarians. Their children are being raised on lacto-ovo-vegetarian, vegan, and macrobiotic diets, respectively.

> I have raised a family of five boys and three girls with the help of my husband on a vegetarian diet of raw and cooked fruits and vegetables and protein from eggs, cheese, peas, beans and nuts. Except for a few slight attacks, they escaped the childhood illnesses prevalent at the time and were in excellent health.

> My daughter has been vegan from birth and is now six and very healthy—apart from the odd cold which she recovers from very quickly. The local doctor admits to her being the healthiest child at his daughter's birthday party. And she has boundless energy without being hyperactive.

> My children eat macrobiotics. They've never eaten animal products and are very, very healthy. My wife and myself were macrobiotic before the children were born so they were raised this way. They have never had dairy products, sugar or honey. My son drinks soy milk. He calls it white juice. It's not a problem. They've never been sick and their bodies are strong.

The general good health of the vegetarian children in our sample contrasts with the grave warnings of relatives and in-laws. Many parents are criticized by others for not feeding their children meat, and some are put under considerable pressure from well-meaning but intrusive family members. A recent reader poll conducted by *Vegetarian Times* magazine tells a similar story: One half of respondents say their relatives are less than enthusiastic about their plans to raise their children as vegetarians. (However, the poll also found that 70 percent of vegetarian parents report receiving support from friends, and two thirds report receiving the support of their pediatricians.)[3] Parents often react to family pressure by reaffirming their commitment to raise their children as vegetarians and by doing everything possible to ensure that their children grow up healthy and happy. The following story from Theresa is typical of many mothers' experiences with relatives:

> I had a few problems with my mother and mother-in-law while I was pregnant. They couldn't understand why I was remaining vegetarian. My mother warned me that if the baby didn't get enough protein, it would be brain damaged. It was statements like that that made me eat so well that my son became too big for natural birth! Our son was totally breastfed for his first six months and people frowned on that too. They also frown now that he is two and not weaned. My obstetrician said being vegetarian is fine, and he was close to being one himself, being of Indian descent. We are bringing our son up as a vegetarian. My husband's mother thinks we are depriving him of so much because we have cut sugar completely out of his life. He enjoys fruit and muffins as candy. My mother is really supportive of the way we are raising him but we have to watch my husband's mother. She tries to feed him cake and cookies (he is only two) and likes to recite nursery rhymes that I hate like, "This little piggy had roast beef."

Before concluding our discussion of health implications for children, we note that three people in our sample had been raised as vegetarians from birth. As noted above, many people think that a vegetarian diet is nutritionally inadequate for growing children. However, our three respondents had all grown into healthy and active adults. Mervyn, a 34-year-old journalist, is an example of the potential of vegetarian children:

> The state of my health? No major illnesses, no major injuries, ever. I've been running marathons, ultramarathons (50 miles), and shorter races (about 30–40 per year) for the past eight years, with no significant physical problems. I've played semi-pro baseball off and on since my late teens. My growth certainly wasn't stunted. At 6′3″, I'm the tallest on record from either side of the family. My brother and sister, also raised as vegetarians from birth, are 6′2″ and 5′10″, respectively. All of us are excellent athletes, noted for stamina, though our parents had no athletic inclination.

Children, of course, have nutritional needs that are greater than those of adults. Consequently, it is important for vegetarian parents, as for all parents, to seek out information and advice on their children's diets. But, as Mervyn's case illustrates, children's nutritional requirements can be adequately met with a meatless diet, provided that adequate care is taken.

Children's Diets

Children have acute senses of smell and taste, and for this reason, tend to prefer simple foods. And they can be finicky eaters, regardless of their family diet. Nevertheless, according to the parents in our sample, young children develop tastes for vegetarian foods, such as soy milk and tofu, with little trouble. Problems are more likely to occur among children who are switched from a meat-centered diet to a vegetarian diet in midstream; those who are raised from birth as vegetarians readily eat most vegetarian foods without complaint. And although meat and junk food are sometimes tempting to them, healthy vegetarian treats, such as fruit, raisins, granola, and nuts, are also appreciated by most children.

Establishing good eating habits in children when they are young can discourage them from developing a taste for junk food. The following quote from Monika, a music promoter and vegan for 22 years, illustrates this point:

> My four-year-old will say, "Oh, I don't want to eat that. It's got sugar in it." They enjoy the food we eat. Meat is never a problem. The 13- and 16-year-olds are tempted by sweets and donuts—things they see other people eating. They'll sneak out and eat those things, but I always know when they do because the next day they will say, "Oh, we're fasting today." It makes them feel unhealthy to eat that stuff. They will also cheat with cheese, but never with meat. They think it is gross.

Adolescents experience strong pressure to conform to their peer groups, and this can conflict with their vegetarian diets in situations where food is shared. To deal with this, some parents make an effort to prepare foods that fit in with adolescents' lifestyles, such as vegetarian burgers and "hot dogs," when other adolescents are around. This helps to avoid embarrassment on the part of their children and minimizes the possibility of teenage rebellion. Serving food that appeals to adolescents requires a certain amount of effort. But as some parents suggested, "keeping up with the kids" is critical in keeping adolescents on the right track. Monika offered some advice on this topic:

> You should supplement their parties with vegetarian burgers and hot dogs because they will want them if they see their friends eating them. When they bring their friends over, give them these foods. Their friends are not going to know the difference; they just think they are eating burgers. With the teenagers, you've got to learn vegetarian recipes and keep the food exciting. You need to make food colorful because you eat with your eyes first. If food is boring, they won't eat it. Try new things, like vegetarian tacos. If they are forced to eat food that they don't like at this stage, they will change later and hate vegetarianism. You've got to keep up with the kids. I'm 45 but they think I'm cool. Some vegetarians get boring and dull and will only listen to new age music. They need to give their kids relevant role models, like Michael Jackson and other people who are vegetarian.

Explaining Vegetarianism to Children

Because the eating habits of vegetarian children are at odds with those of most of their peers and the larger society, most parents find it necessary to discuss vegetarianism with their children from an early age. They feel that their children must not only learn what they should and shouldn't eat, but need to understand the reasons and values that underlie their diets. This is necessary if children are to avoid eating meat in situations when it is offered to them and parents are not around to provide guidance. Children must also learn to feel comfortable with and proud of their diets because they are certain to be questioned, and perhaps ridiculed, by others.

However, the extent to which children are able to understand depends very much on their ages. It is unlikely that young children will have the intellectual ability to fully grasp the significance of vegetarianism or even to clearly understand the categories of "animal food" and "plant food." The following story from Valerie, a nutritionist and vegan for 12 years, illustrates this point:

> I have one child aged four. She sometimes gets the health aspects and the ethical aspects of vegetarianism confused. When she was not quite two she wanted to know what type of dead animal candy was.

Some parents make a deliberate effort to educate their children whereas others prefer to answer questions as they arise. Health-oriented parents generally tell their children how much healthier and stronger they are on a meatless diet as opposed to one based on flesh. For parents who are ethical vegetarians, it is difficult to know how much to tell children about factory farms and slaughterhouses. Many adults feel burdened by this knowledge, and young children would undoubtedly be distressed at hearing the whole truth. Consequently, many parents explain these matters in general terms but leave out the more upsetting details.

> My children, aged 5, 4 and almost 3, have never had meat, fish, or poultry. Or sugar. I haven't run into any problems

yet. My oldest will be starting school this fall, so I'm sure situations will arise. So far, I've explained to them that animals are our friends so we don't eat them. I've tried to explain how our lives are all related, whether human, animal, or plant, and I hope a real respect for life will evolve or develop in them.

Most children appear to accept their parents' reasons for being vegetarian—in spite of conflicting views presented by the media, teachers, relatives, and other children. Surprisingly, even very young children often find the notion of not eating animals to be understandable and are cooperative. One mother told us how her young daughter, who had eaten meat now and then when visiting relatives, reacted when the idea of vegetarianism was first explained to her:

When she was two and one-half, I sat down with her and explained that meat was made out of dead animals and I felt it was wrong to eat it. She stopped asking for it immediately and hasn't eaten any since. In fact, the very next time she went to my mother's house, my daughter told her that she didn't eat meat anymore because it was a dead animal. She learned to say "vegetarian" when she was three, and she surprised me one day in the grocery store when a lady was handing out sausage samples and she said, "No thanks. I'm a vegetarian." She is very proud of being vegetarian and doesn't mind at all being different. She has assured me that when she grows up she is going to teach people not to eat animals.

What about the child's point of view? Ronald, aged 11, seemed to be adapting well to a vegetarian diet and lifestyle. As he told us:

My family are strict vegetarians. I like being vegetarian because it makes me healthy and strong and good in my school work, and I am creative. I paint and color a lot. We are peace loving people. We don't hurt animals. Eating vegetables makes us peace loving.

Nine year old Alisa is another example of a child who was strongly committed to vegetarianism—in spite of occasional problems in sharing pizzas with her friends. As she said:

> I have been a vegetarian all my life. I know my Mom likes it, for she is vegetarian too. It's tempting though. My friends have sleepovers and usually they go out for pizza. Well, that's okay, but with pepperoni and anchovies I feel funny picking it out of the pizza, but I do. But I'm never going to give up being a vegetarian.

Parental Strictness

The question of whether or not children should be completely forbidden to eat meat is a difficult one for many vegetarian parents. Some feel pressured by relatives to let their children eat meat occasionally. Others live with meat-eating spouses who not only set a conflicting example, but often insist that the children be fed meat. And others worry that if they are too restrictive, eating meat will seem especially desirable—like forbidden fruit. How demanding should parents be? Parents arrive at different answers to this question.

In our sample, 70 percent of parents are raising their children on completely vegetarian diets; the remaining 30 percent allow their children to eat meat to some degree. Interestingly, these results are similar to those reported in a 1987 poll conducted by *Vegetarian Times* magazine. In this poll, 33 percent of vegetarian parents said they would allow their children to eat hot dogs at a birthday party.[4]

The 30 percent in our sample who allow their children to eat meat do so for one of three reasons. First, some became vegetarian after their children had already been partly raised on meat. These parents felt uncomfortable forcing their decisions on their children. Instead, they hoped that by setting a good example, their children would eventually voluntarily give up meat. Martina, a vegetarian for one year, adopted this strategy:

> If we go to a relative's house and animal flesh is served, I let them eat what they wish. When we go to a restaurant, I let the children order whatever they like, but recently they have been sticking to grilled cheese sandwiches without my prompting. I am not certain how to go about teaching them about vegetarianism, especially since I only made the

> switch myself recently. I am proceeding cautiously and avoiding lectures and proselytizing at the table. If the 5-year-old asks a direct question like, "Why don't you eat meat?" I give her a simple, basic answer without preaching or being overly negative. I would like my children to be enlightened and sympathetic, and I feel, at this point, the best way to accomplish this is by nonhysterical example. I want my children to grow up questioning and thinking for themselves. If they grow up thinking critically and decide that Mom's wrong, then so be it.

Second, some vegetarian parents allow their children to eat meat because they live with meat-eating spouses and the children's diet is an issue of disagreement. Interestingly, when vegetarian men are married to meat-eating women, the children are usually raised as vegetarians. However, when vegetarian women are married to meat-eating men, the children are usually not raised as vegetarians—which says something about the relative power of men and women in our society. In some families, this leads to outright conflict. But even in families in which compromises are reached, parents often feel as if they are competing for their children's allegiance. And if the child decides to follow one parent's example, it sometimes causes resentment on the part of the other parent. Bernice found it necessary to walk a fine line in trying to be fair to everyone in her household:

> I have an 8-month-old baby. She eats chicken and turkey baby food now, and once in a while some beef. Her doctor felt she should have some kind of meat once a day, so I'm following that advice although I wish it were otherwise. My husband just doesn't want me to keep meat from her, and he would rather that I don't tell her that it is wrong to eat meat. But he knows that I feel that way, and I can't say otherwise. I'll tell her that I hope she agrees with me that it is wrong but not to blame Daddy for what he is taught. My husband knows that I'll exert a strong influence on her and that is OK, as long as I give her no absolutes, allowing her the final decision. I believe that this is the best approach.

Third, some parents are concerned that their children will feel left out in social situations. Accordingly, they allow their children to deviate from their usual vegetarian diets on such occasions. As one mother said:

> My three year old son is a vegetarian at home, but eats meat if he is offered it at someone else's home. I do not stop this because I don't want him to feel left out or deprived. I feel that when he is old enough, he will automatically reject meat.

One vegan mother reached a similar compromise by allowing her child to use dairy products when away from home:

> She is an avowed vegetarian at home, and although she adores cow's milk and cheese when she can get it at preschool, she's more than willing to avoid meat and eggs. It's a paradox. We let her have dairy when we're out so she'll feel less odd, but we never realized that she would like it so much.

Parents realize that even if raised as vegetarians, their children will have many opportunities to eat meat as they get older. The starting of school, in particular, is a time when many vegetarian parents feel anxiety about their children's diets. They are aware that children can be cruel and can exert a great deal of pressure to conform. In the face of this, most parents feel that the best they can do is to instill a sense of ethics in their children, set a good example, and hope that their children see the value of a consistently vegetarian way of life. Many expect that their children will eat meat now and then, but feel that their children will have to make up their own minds. Most of the parents who think this way believe their children will ultimately make the right decision. Douglas, who was raising his children on a vegetarian macrobiotic diet, put it this way:

> As time goes on they'll start to pal around with their peers and see other foods, and we're just going to let that happen. We hope they've had a good start, and we'll try to educate them along the way. But they need to see it for themselves. The example at home is the first step that needs to be taken. If we feel strong and stay with our diet, I don't think it will be hard for our children to stay with it.

On the other hand, some parents feel that eating flesh is clearly and completely wrong, either for ethical or health-related reasons. Consequently, the question of "choice" for their children is not relevant. Two parents, one a health vegetarian and the other an ethical vegetarian, made the following comments:

> People would question what we are doing with our son such as, "Aren't you going to give him a choice about meat?" I tell them, "He will eventually have the choice to smoke cigarettes, but I'm not going to offer him one now."

> My children will be raised as vegans. None of this philosophy about letting them make their own choices. Deliberate cruelty and unnecessary killing aren't choices, they're crimes.

Regardless of how strictly they are raised, the question of what children eat as they grow older and become more independent is a source of continuing concern for many vegetarian parents. The following quote from Marina illustrates what must be every vegetarian parent's nightmare:

> About a year ago my daughter (8 years old) said, "Mommy, I'm going to be just like you when I grow up." How nice, I thought. "Yup," she went on, "I'm going to eat meat and lots of sugar, watch TV all day long, live in a regular house in the city, drive around a lot in a big car, and use lots of electricity." "What?" I asked. "Well, you do exactly the opposite of what your mother did, so I'm going to be the exact opposite of you," she said.

Problems for Vegetarian Children

Few parents are worried about health problems or nutritional deficiencies in their children. The biggest concern of parents is that their children will be ridiculed by other kids for being different. This is, in fact, a common problem; about one third of parents say their children experience social difficulties because of their meatless diets. However, according to parents, most children cope with these situations reasonably well and are not too upset. The following boy, whose parents are members of the

International Society for Krishna Consciousness, adapted well to life in a new school:

> He started going to a new school. When he began eating his lunch the other kids teased him and tested him. "What are you eating?" they asked. "Why don't you have a bologna sandwich or something normal?" He told them, "I'm a vegetarian and these are chickpeas and potatoes. They make you strong. See?" And he showed them his muscles. He happens to be big for his age and smart—he skipped a grade. So all the kids respected him even though he was a vegetarian.

Some parents mention that their children coped better in some parts of the country than in others. Clearly, some schools and neighborhoods are more supportive than others for vegetarian children. One mother found that a move from Chicago to the Midwest cut her daughter off from her support group of vegetarian friends:

> She likes being vegetarian, but it was easier when we lived in Chicago because we had a lot of vegan and vegetarian friends. Here it is not so supportive. She is in school with children who go to McDonald's and sometimes she feels a little bit out of it. We strive to be supportive and to listen well.

Some children deal with social pressure better than others, and the child's personality is a factor in whether or not being "different" is a problem. In general, some children cope with stress better than others—for reasons that are still largely unclear to psychologists. The comments of the following vegetarian mother reveal a resilient child who is not worried by the fact that she is unlike her agemates:

> My daughter (6 years old) has a strong personality which helps her a lot, as we live in the middle of a farming community and are still considered strange for not eating meat and stranger still for not eating dairy products. She copes very well at school where she is the only child to take a packed lunch every day. She couldn't care less what people think. I give her a lot of credit.

Major personality differences can also occur between siblings. The following story from Ramona indicates that even within the same family, some children cope better than others with social pressure:

> Our two girls were ages 3 and 6 when they were put into a new eating lifestyle with us. The younger one has no memory of eating meat. She has adjusted much better than the older girl, being more assertive and aggressive in nature. She never hides the fact that she is vegetarian. In fact, she proudly states it. However, the older one was much more affected by peer pressure and the remarks made to her. So in her middle years, she ceased to openly admit that she didn't eat meat. They both ardently believe in the things we taught them and did not "cheat" because of it. We always told them that if they decide to be like other people and eat meat, we would not make them feel guilty. They are now 18 and 21—still vegetarian and out in the open about it.

The following story from a man raised as a vegetarian also demonstrates that the responses of individual children within the same family can differ considerably:

> My younger brother has always been more susceptible to peer pressure generally, and he did get a lot of flak for being vegetarian. He became a meat eater as soon as he left home at 18. My sister, ten years younger, has joined me in remaining vegetarian. Interestingly, the more successful my brother becomes in business, the less meat he eats. It is as if he no longer has to prove himself.

How do people raised as vegetarians evaluate their childhoods? Those with whom we spoke were generally positive in spite of the problems that they encountered. Carolyn, who was raised as a vegetarian in England, commented:

> When I was a little girl, I would tell my schoolteachers or anyone else who asked about my vegetarian ways that "animals are my friends." Once, another small girl said if I did not eat at least one spoonful of meat in my life, I would die—but my mother put me right. Later on at boarding school at age 9, I would pretend to be ill just so that I could

> stay in bed all day, because I never got sick. Being the only vegetarian at school, I sometimes went hungry, but I never thought about it. Throughout my school life I never got teased about my vegetarian beliefs, which I put down to my physical strength which brought me a lot of respect.

Avoiding Problems

With a little foresight, vegetarian parents can avoid many of the awkward social situations their children might face. For example, most parents find that it is possible to arrange meatless snacks for their children at preschool. When children get older, parents usually have to prepare lunches for them to take to school. Although parents find that this requires more effort on their part, it also means that their children are eating better-quality food than are their classmates; many school cafeterias continue to serve hot dogs, hamburgers, pizza, french fries, soft drinks, and other foods that have little nutritional value.

As a general rule, parents need to be careful to make sure teachers and caretakers understand their children's diets in some detail if slipups are to be prevented. Parents should not assume that people who are looking after their children will understand what the term "vegetarian" includes. Some parents mention that preschool teachers or others had fed chicken, fish, gelatin, eggs, dairy products, or other foods to their children under the assumption that they were acceptable.

When children go to parties, it is usually necessary to arrange vegetarian food in advance. Some parents send food with their children if they think the host is unwilling or unlikely to provide vegetarian food. Sometimes these arrangements work well, and sometimes they do not, as the following quotes illustrate:

> When my children are invited to parties, I talk with the mother about whether it would be possible to have my children bring a nondairy cupcake and have tofutti instead of eating cake and ice cream. So far, the mothers have been gracious towards me.

> Recently the girls were invited to a party and when I phoned with an R.S.V.P., I explained the situation about food. She assured me that everything would be OK. When the time came, I discovered that the refreshments consisted of hot dogs and soda pop. She ended up making peanut butter sandwiches and orange juice for my daughters. It was an unnecessarily embarrassing situation for all of us.

In Australia and England, girls—and sometimes boys—do cookery classes at school. And in the United States, children may cook meals as part of home economics courses. These classes can create situations that conflict with vegetarian family values if meat is involved. (In addition to cooking classes, conflict can arise for vegetarian children who are expected to participate in biology class dissections.) One Australian mother was worried about how she was going to deal with this situation:

> Cookery classes at school will become a problem next year. I don't know whether to say nothing and let her cook a meat meal or whether to back her up and insist she doesn't participate on meat cookery days. The latter course seems to cause a lot of hassles for an eleven year old. Kids that age can be damaged by having to take alternative lines from their contemporaries, especially controversial ones.

Home–school conflicts, in which teachers require children to engage in activities their parents do not approve of, are not exclusive to vegetarians. Some parents do not want their children to be exposed to sex education; others do not want their children to learn about evolutionary theory or Marxist ideas; and others do not want their children to say the pledge of allegiance to the flag. Whether children should be expected to participate in school activities that clash with family values is a decision that parents and children should discuss together, but the decision is not always easy.

Most vegetarian parents realize that their children may be exposed to pressure, or even ridicule, from their peers. However, in most cases, children and adolescents do not base their friendship choices on things as minor as bringing a sack lunch to school every day or passing up the occasional hot dog. Furthermore, children who learn that one set of standards is expected at home and a different set is allowed elsewhere are likely to conclude that "right and wrong" simply depend on the situation. If children are to internalize a set of values, they should be expected to behave consistently.

Long-Term Prospects for Vegetarian Children

Do vegetarian children remain vegetarian for life? Parents' concerns that their children will revert to eating meat in adulthood are sometimes fulfilled, although this is not always seen as a bad thing. Many people raised as vegetarians need to go through a period of eating flesh to find out for themselves what it is like. But most of these lapses are short-lived, and the majority of vegetarian children appear to become vegetarians in adulthood. Often, a period of meat-eating helps to reinforce their commitment to vegetarianism in later life. The following stories from parents illustrate this trend:

> My 16-year-old son resisted because of pure teenage rebellion. But he is now feeling it in his own heart and making the change for his own reasons. My daughter is a vegan and is a fine example of glowing health and happiness.
>
> My daughter was three years old when we joined the Seventh-Day Adventist Church. So, she had meat for three years and was tuned in to it. In fact, during a couple of her teenage years she went back to eating meat. My son was born after we became vegetarian, and you couldn't get him to touch it with a ten foot pole. He thinks it is repugnant. However, our daughter is vegetarian again and is raising her children as vegetarian.

Most parents whose children have reached adulthood comment that their children experienced some inconvenience in being raised as vegetarians. However, they also feel that their children benefited in many ways—not only in terms of health, but in terms of character. Overall, the benefits are thought to outweigh the costs.

> It was a tough road to hoe for the children. But if I had to do it all over again, I'd do it exactly the same way. They had some crosses to bear, but I believe they are better off for it and understand human nature and its cruelties in a way most people don't.
>
> Our children have stuck to vegetarianism and are all active in the animal rights movement. I believe that they have received great psychological benefits from living out their love for animals without the disharmony that I once experienced.

It appears, from the comments above, that most children are resilient and adapt to a vegetarian diet and lifestyle without major problems. Clearly, vegetarian parents should not worry that they are imposing an onerous duty on their children. Instead, they might just find that their children are entirely comfortable with, and even enthusiastic about, living as vegetarians.

Chapter 8

Conclusions and Recommendations

How does vegetarianism stack up? After adopting meatless diets, the great majority of people report improvements in health, including increases in stamina and energy level, the alleviation of earlier health problems, fewer colds, improvements in complexion, decreases in weight, and more regular bowel movements. Psychological benefits are also the rule and include less guilt, an increase in self-esteem, an enhanced sense of morality, feeling less aggressive, feeling more compassionate, an increase in sense of self-control, and greater emotional stability. In addition, many people feel more spiritual after eliminating flesh from their diets. In the light of all these benefits, vegetarianism stands out as a viable and positive lifestyle for the majority of people who embrace it.

However, as we have seen, the road to vegetarianism is not always smooth, and most people encounter practical problems along the way. Many individuals have a difficult time adjusting to vegetarianism. Some have cravings for meat that last for months or even years; others don't know what to cook and wind up with monotonous, boring diets. Most vegetarians experience difficulty when eating out and traveling. And conflict between job expectations and vegetarian beliefs and practices is not uncommon.

Social problems also occur. Resistance from families and friends is the rule for new vegetarians; many, in fact, find they lose old friends during the transition. And dealing with new acquaintances is difficult as one contends with constant criticism, ridicule, and interrogation. Vegetarianism reduces some people's love lives to lost causes. It can also come between husbands and wives, and in extreme cases, can lead to divorce.

Given this list of potential pitfalls, one might wonder if the benefits are worth the effort. The answer to this question is clearly "Yes," according to the great majority of vegetarians with whom we spoke. All but one or two felt their lives had been improved and enriched by giving up animal flesh, and virtually all wished to remain vegetarian for the rest of their lives. None regretted the experience. (Of course, the people in our sample are those who survived the transition; an unknown but probably substantial number of people "drop out" and return to flesh-eating. We will have more to say on these people later.)

Vegetarianism can be a nuisance. But it is clear that the major difficulties in vegetarians' lives are generated, not by the diet itself, but by the complexity of living as a herbivore in a meat-eating society. These problems are frustrating, of course, but the fact that they are primarily social in nature should be a cause for optimism for vegetarians, because people can change. Without doubt, as individuals are educated about the benefits of eliminating—or at least cutting down—their consumption of meat, social attitudes will become more accepting and the lives of vegetarians will become easier.

However, the realization that the situation is gradually improving is little comfort for those who are currently experiencing difficulties in their lives. Accordingly, we offer a few recommendations for making life a little easier. Some of our comments are aimed at people who would like to stop eating meat but haven't yet taken the first step. Other points are appropriate for those who have recently given up meat and are experiencing the ups and downs of the transition period. And a few are for those who have comfortably settled into the vegetarian lifestyle but still experience the occasional bump or two. We base our suggestions on three sources: first, the collective experiences of the more than 300 vegetarians in our study; second, our knowledge of psychological techniques useful for helping people to make other lifestyle changes, such as giving up smoking, controlling overeating, and maintaining exercise programs; and third, our discussions with people who stopped being vegetarian for various reasons.

GETTING STARTED

Any major change in behavior, including a change in one's diet, consists of three stages: making a decision, changing the behavior, and maintaining that change.

Making the Decision

Decisions require information, and as a rule, the better the quality of the information on which a decision is made, the better the decision. Vegetarianism is no exception. The first thing people should do if they are seriously contemplating eliminating meat from their diets is to learn as much as they can. Most large libraries contain books on vegetarianism (a list of useful references is provided on pages 268–269), and a good deal of reading material can be obtained from vegetarian societies and organizations. Other vegetarians, of course, are worth talking to, although one should keep in mind that considerable variation in beliefs and practices exists among individuals.

Gathering information is critical for several reasons. First, information is necessary to clarify one's motives. Many people take a long time to stop eating meat because their initial reasons are vague. And a lack of clarity and commitment to one's beliefs can lead novice vegetarians to abandon the effort and return to meat-eating as soon as the going gets tough. People who do some preliminary research, however, discover a variety of sound reasons for minimizing their consumption of animal flesh. Consequently, as they learn more, their motives become clearer and their commitment to change becomes stronger. Psychological studies show that behavior change is easier and occurs more quickly if individuals strongly believe in what they are doing than if they are uncertain. So it is important in the early stages to be clear about one's motives.

Second, information is necessary to deal with nutritional questions that may occur. A good deal of dietary misinformation exists in our society, and many people have distorted views about the consequences of vegetarian diets. Earlier, we saw that many individuals are anxious when they first stop eating meat because they are uninformed about nutrition. However, as we pointed out, there are no nutritional risks associated with a well-balanced diet that excludes animal flesh. A little preliminary knowledge on this topic would take away the edge of anxiety in the minds of many people as they embark on their new diets. (Medical doctors may not be the best people to approach for information as few are trained in nutrition. Vegetarian registered dieticians can be located through an organization called VEGEDINE; its address is provided on page 267.)

Third, information is crucial if one is to deal with the questions, criticisms, and arguments of others. As we saw earlier, many vegetarians find that the initial reactions of new acquaintances are negative. It is an unpleasant fact of life, but most vegetarians have to deal with occasional challenges to their beliefs. However, having a few facts on hand makes it easier to deal with these situations. And because the facts are persuasive, an informed response can earn the grudging respect of many critics.

Fourth, and on a more positive note, vegetarians are often asked questions by people who are genuinely interested. By being informed, vegetarians can provide information and serve as positive sources of change within their social circles.

Making the Change

As we have seen, some people successfully make the transition from omnivore to herbivore overnight. However, most people find it easier to become vegetarian by making a gradual transition over a period of several months. For those who take the gradual approach—and we assume that most people do—we suggest the following procedures.

First, set yourself a series of small goals. The final goal, of course, is to eliminate animal flesh from your diet. But this is a major long-term goal, and most people find it easier to work with a series of smaller goals that can be accomplished in shorter periods of time. The first step might be very simple, for example, getting through one day without eating meat. The second step might be getting through one weekend without eating meat. And the third step might involve extending the time period to an entire week. The precise time periods are not critical. The important point is to formulate the goals you want to achieve, along with a realistic timetable for achieving them. Two or three months to complete the transition might be a reasonable period for some people; six months to a year might be better for others.

Reward yourself as each small goal is achieved. This can be done by taking something you enjoy doing—such as going to a movie, buying new clothes, or going out to eat—and making it contingent on achieving your goal. For example, if your goal is to go one week without eating any red meat or chicken, and you succeed, then treat yourself to a movie on the weekend. But only reward yourself if you succeed. If you are a film buff, your desire to see the latest movie everyone is talking about will increase your motivation to achieve your goal.

These goals might apply to all forms of animal flesh simultaneously. Alternatively, you can start with red meat, followed by chicken, followed by fish—or any other order that makes sense to you. Whatever your goals are, it is important to keep them flexible. For example, if your cousin from out of state shows up for a week, your program can be temporarily interrupted. Just get back on track again when events are favorable.

Another useful technique is to monitor your daily behavior by allocating points for achieving small goals. For example, you might give yourself a point every time you get through a meal without eating meat, making it possible to earn up to three points per day. Enter your daily points on a calendar and total them up at the end of every week. An important aspect of this procedure is that you do this for the week prior to changing your diet; this will indicate your baseline meat consumption. Then continue keeping track after you begin to eliminate meat; this will show how effective you have been in changing your behavior over time. You might, for example, have a baseline of 7 points before changing your diet, and achieve 12 points during the first week, 15 points during the second week, and 19 points during the third week. Now and then you might have a bad week during which your total drops. This is to be expected. But your weekly totals should present a gradually rising pattern.

This technique focuses your attention on your behavior at every meal; after all, each one is worth one point. In addition, the technique supplies an extra incentive for avoiding meat: believe it or not, people love to accumulate points. You can also increase the incentive value of your points by "cashing" them in for certain privileges; for example, 20 points might be exchanged for a meal out at a restaurant—vegetarian, of course.

After you have been modifying your diet for a while, expect a few cravings for meat. This is perfectly normal. But if you give in to your cravings, don't feel that you have failed. It is natural and common to eat meat again after you have begun to think of yourself as a vegetarian. Simply note what you have done and then get on with making the transition; don't get sidetracked from the larger goal.

Meat can be tempting to the novice vegetarian, but steps can be taken to minimize this problem. First, avoid situations in which you might be tempted. If you are going to a party or a social gathering, eat something first so you won't feel like nibbling on meat-based snacks. Alternatively, if appropriate, bring some vegetarian food with you. It is also a good idea to carry some food when you are traveling. On the open road it is often difficult to find a place to eat where everything on the menu isn't dripping with grease. If you are going out to eat with friends, suggest a place where you know you will be able to order something vegetarian. Most of the time people are waiting for a suggestion anyway, so it might as well come from you. Finally, if you get cravings for a hamburger or a hot dog, eat a soyburger or a tofu hot dog instead. Textured vegetable protein products have the same texture and appearance as meat, and many people discover they satisfy cravings for familiar foods.

If cravings for meat are a persistent problem, a good way to deal with them is through the use of mental imagery. Imagine an extremely unpleasant scene involving meat. For example, think of a dead pet cooked and lying on a serving platter. Visualize your arteries clogging up with thick waxy plaque and your heart struggling to force blood through them. See a piece of rancid meat on your plate with worms crawling through it. Or think of a large vein protruding from a steak and spurting out blood. Find an image that works well for you, and when a craving occurs, conjure up the image in your mind. Not surprisingly, most people find this technique is sufficient to depress their appetite for meat.

You can also use imagery in positive ways. Think of images that reflect beneficial outcomes of vegetarianism. For example, visualize your strong heart pumping blood through arteries as smooth as glass. Imagine yourself petting farm animals, such as lambs and calves, and telling them that you're their friend. Think of tropical rain forests in Brazil that will be spared as the demand for beef in the West declines. These images should help to strengthen your resolve to forgo that cheeseburger.

Before concluding this section, we would like to add one qualification: Individuals should not attempt a vegetarian diet if they have eating disorders. Eating disorders, such as anorexia nervosa (extremely low consumption of calories) and bulimia (uncontrollable eating), are most commonly found among adolescent and young adult females. People with these problems are excessively preoccupied with food, and a switch to a meatless diet may aggravate these problems. We spoke with several women who became vegetarian while suffering from eating disorders. As one person said:

> The most notable act of self-abuse I performed was to go on eating binges during which I added to my sense of guilt by eating meat, and then condemned myself for my evilness in doing so. It was inevitable that, once the eating disorder became active, I would consume meat. It was equally inevitable that I would indulge in horrible recriminations for weeks afterward.

We strongly recommend that people with eating disorders seek professional help. The adoption of a vegetarian diet should only be attempted once the problem is well under control.

MINIMIZING SOCIAL CONFLICT

Some vegetarians find that their families and circles of friends approve of their new lifestyles and are supportive. These people are lucky. As we found earlier, tension is common between vegetarians and their meat-eating families and friends, at least initially. Although it is impossible to completely eliminate the friction generated by incompatible lifestyles, it is possible in most cases to smooth over disagreements, avoid embarrassment, and keep relations cordial.

Before getting into specifics, there are two general rules to keep in mind: First, don't make people defensive about their eating habits, and second, don't lead people to believe that you are deliberately trying to change their beliefs or behavior (even if you are). All things being equal, people are easiest to deal with if they feel comfortable around you and don't think that you are forcing your views on them. Under these conditions, people are also maximally receptive to new ideas—a point we return to later.

Many parents and other family members are sincerely concerned about what they perceive to be health risks associated with a meatless diet. In these cases, parents' minds can be put at ease by giving them a book or pamphlet on vegetarian nutrition (vegetarian societies can help you find a good one). Demonstrating that you have a responsible attitude toward nutrition by eating sensibly also helps.

In other cases, parents' objections are based on the perception that vegetarianism represents a rejection of their beliefs and values. When this occurs, vegetarians should point out that certain information was not available 5, 10, or 20 years ago. For example, the medical research linking consumption of a high-cholesterol, high-fat, low-fiber diet to coronary heart disease and cancer was only compiled relatively recently. Twenty years ago, most people thought beef was a health food. Similarly, it has only been within the last few decades that modern "animal factories" have replaced the traditional family farm, and knowledge of the abuses involved in these new modes of production has only recently come to public attention. And awareness of our serious environmental problems—many of which are linked to cattle grazing and livestock production—has only emerged in the last couple of decades.

Given these changes, it is clear that people in the West need to modify their eating habits, and that the standard diet of earlier decades is not the diet best suited for the future. In other words, becoming vegetarian does not involve a rejection of the past, but adapting to present and future realities. Putting things into this sort of perspective may help to keep parents from feeling a personal rejection.

Although parents often react critically, they generally become supportive after a year or two. This is partly because they discover that their children are still healthy and happy even though they don't eat meat. In the meantime, vegetarians can help to keep family relations harmonious by seeing to it that their diets result in minimal disruption of traditional family activities. It is important, in particular, that vegetarians continue to sit at the dinner table with their families and share meals. This can be facilitated if vegetarians offer to cook and bring food of their own to family gatherings. They can also expose their families to recipes, ethnic styles of cooking, and alternative vegetarian foods.

Our results show that many people lose friends after adopting a fleshless diet. As we stated earlier, it is important not to put your friends on the defensive by attacking their eating habits. Instead, do as much as you reasonably can to make them feel comfortable in your presence—particularly when eating. But if eating together makes them (or you) uneasy, then replace activities centered around dining with other pursuits, such as walking, visiting the beach, seeing films, or going out to hear music.

Most people, of course, vary to some extent from year to year in their attitudes, beliefs, and behavior, and good friends continually adapt to each others' changes. A strong friendship will survive a change to vegetarianism, just as it will survive most other changes. But if your friends stop inviting you around, or if they refuse your invitations, the inevitable should be accepted philosophically. If the main thing you and your friends had in common was chewing on chicken bones, then perhaps you weren't such good friends after all. Don't forget that it is not difficult to meet new people and make new friends—preferably individuals who are tolerant of vegetarians or are vegetarians themselves.

We found that new acquaintances often react negatively to vegetarianism, and some are openly critical. However, you should not get drawn into arguments with these people—unless you really want to. Remember, you are under no obligation to justify your views or behavior to anyone. In fact, little is achieved in many of these debates. Some people, for example, are simply argumentative and are not really interested in a serious exchange of views. Others may be open-minded, but if you adopt a confrontational manner, and if you force them to publicly declare their opposition to vegetarianism, you make it more difficult for them to change later.

Unless you are the type who loves a good debate, we suggest you try to keep the discussion on the light side. A little bit of humor can go a long way in minimizing tension. For example, a person once said to us, "Why do you eat vegetables? They have feelings like animals do." At this point we could have launched into a detailed and impassioned argument for the existence of pain in animals but not in plants. Instead, our response was, "Oh yeah? When was the last time you took your cabbage for a walk?" At this, he laughed and said, "Well, you've got a point." By using humor, the error in his argument was exposed, he didn't feel threatened, and a seed was planted that may someday lead him to think more seriously about the issue.

In dealing with others, you should also be prepared for questions about your use of leather or other animal products. People who ask these questions hope to expose inconsistencies in your behavior or beliefs. Consequently, if you are an ethical vegetarian, you should attempt to be as consistent as possible in this regard. This isn't fair, of course. After all, how many people are interrogated about other moral decisions, such as decisions to be honest or to be nice to children? Vegetarians are often singled out, and that's an unpleasant fact of life.

But it is a good idea to be one step ahead of the interrogators. Ethical vegetarians should be able to describe the other nondietary changes they have made in order to attain consistency, for example, in purchasing alternatives to leather products when they are available, and in using cruelty-free personal care products (that is, products that contain no animal ingredients and are not tested on animals). Vegetarians should also feel comfortable in pointing out that alternatives are often *not* available; for example, it may be impossible to find nonleather briefcases. If you are not an ethical vegetarian, your situation is easier, but you will still be expected to provide a clear explanation for why you use leather or other animal products.

Social conflict over diet is most difficult when it occurs between spouses. As we found earlier, it is not uncommon for vegetarian wives to have meat-eating husbands. In these situations, there are four outcomes. First, one spouse converts the other. Second, the situation degenerates into an impasse in which both partners refuse to change, with constant tension being the result. Third, the partners split up or divorce. And fourth, a workable and mutually satisfying compromise is found. Outcome one is the preferred one for most vegetarians—assuming that the vegetarian converts the meat-eater—but outcome four is more common.

Compromises that work are those in which the meat-eating spouse (usually the husband) agrees not to eat meat at home, but continues to eat meat when dining out at restaurants or with friends and family. Compromises can also be arranged in which meat-eating spouses cook their own meat meals. This arrangement works as an occasional variation; however, it is unsatisfying on a daily basis because of the inconvenience involved in preparing two dishes at every meal.

Arrangements that do not work well are those in which the vegetarian spouse (usually the wife) is compelled to cook meat for her husband even though she does not eat it herself. If a wife feels comfortable cooking meat for her husband, then this may not be a problem. But usually there is some resentment, and this can have a negative impact on the long-term quality of the marital relationship.

In our opinion, if a husband insists that his wife cook meat, she has several good reasons for refusing. For one thing, it is insensitive to ask vegetarians to cook animal flesh if it makes them feel uneasy. More importantly, it is unethical to coerce people into violating their beliefs. Vegetarians need to draw a line somewhere, and this is an appropriate place. Besides, it is fair to expect that husbands pitch in and do their share of the cooking; if they want to eat meat, there is nothing stopping them from cooking it themselves. All in all, it is probably better for the relationship in the long run if the vegetarian sticks to her guns and expects some compromise on the part of her spouse.

CHANGING PEOPLE'S ATTITUDES

Because vegetarians often find themselves discussing their diets with others, and because many wish to spread their knowledge about the benefits of decreasing meat consumption, we include nine suggestions for changing the attitudes and behavior of others. These principles are derived from general research on attitude change conducted by psychologists, but they have been adapted for the topic at hand.

First, when trying to change someone's attitudes or behavior, divide your larger goal into a series of smaller ones. Don't expect to convert a steak-lover into a tofu-eater overnight. Instead, try to persuade the person to try a vegetarian meal now and then, or to cut down on red meat. Similarly, don't expect to turn a cattle rancher into an animal rights activist. Instead, get the person to read an article on farm animal reform. This is sometimes called the "foot-in-the-door" technique: People are more likely to comply with a large request if they have first complied with a small request. Once the first step is taken, it becomes more difficult for the person to refuse later requests.

Second, as we have already noted, be informed about vegetarianism. When dealing with others, your perceived competence on the topic is your most important resource. Few people will be persuaded by a person who doesn't understand any of the fundamentals of nutrition or factory farming.

Third, tailor your approach to fit the person. For example,

people who are concerned about fitness are more receptive to arguments dealing with health, while people who are animal lovers are more receptive to arguments dealing with ethical issues. Find the person's area of interest and present your points accordingly.

Fourth, be a good role model. As we found earlier, many people are first persuaded to give up meat after being introduced to a vegetarian whom they admire. It is important to show the world that vegetarians are healthy, happy, well-adjusted people. In addition, point to other positive role models who are vegetarian: historical figures, writers, or popular entertainers.

Fifth, find some basis of similarity with the person you are trying to persuade. In general, people respond more to similar than to dissimilar others. If they think you have nothing in common with them, they may find your arguments irrelevant; but if they discover you share certain things—such as a concern with fitness, a political orientation, or an interest in the stock market—they will be more likely to listen carefully to what you have to say. Emphasize points of agreement with the other person.

Sixth, discuss the issues with meat-eaters when they are alone. If you tackle a group of meat-eaters all at once, they will close ranks, reinforce, and support each other. But if you get them on a one-to-one basis, they may be relatively receptive to what you have to say.

Seventh, always stress the personal benefits of vegetarianism. Intellectual arguments and altruistic motives are important, but people also need to anticipate personal rewards before they will change. Informing individuals that vegetarian food is delicious and good for their waistlines provides extra incentives to give it a try.

Eighth, don't put people on the defensive. As we noted earlier, a confrontational strategy forces individuals into a position contrary to yours and gives them an opportunity to think of and rehearse antivegetarian arguments. This is particularly problematic if there is an audience; when people publicly declare their opposition to vegetarianism, it is difficult for them to change their positions later. Keep your discussions on a friendly level as much as possible.

Ninth, don't try too hard. If people feel you are deliberately trying to convert them, they will freeze up and resist your persuasion attempts. Individuals don't like to be manipulated. Plant seeds; don't hit people over the head with the message.

LAPSED VEGETARIANS: LESSONS TO BE LEARNED

For the great majority of people, becoming a vegetarian is seen as a lifelong commitment. Unfortunately, things don't always work out this way. Although we don't know precisely how often it occurs, it is not uncommon for vegetarians to revert back to flesh-eating. To explore this topic, we spoke with 25 people who had been vegetarians for a period of time before they returned to earlier eating habits. Some of these individuals became vegetarians again at a later point in time; others did not. Why do people like these give up and go back to a practice they think of as unhealthy, unappealing, or unethical?

Some might think that people who return to meat-eating don't have much of a commitment to vegetarianism in the first place. Although this is true in some cases, it is by no means true in all. In fact, some ex-vegetarians have strong ethical–social reasons for abstaining from flesh and are highly motivated. When it comes to being vegetarian, good intentions are sometimes not enough.

Lack of Social Support

The most common problem is a lack of support from others. A typical situation is one in which people have no vegetarian friends and are entirely dependent on meat-eaters for companionship and social interaction. As we noted earlier, friends and family members tend to react negatively to new vegetarians, and ridicule, criticism, and outright hostility are common. With no fellow vegetarians to offer support or serve as positive role models, isolated vegetarians can come to see their beliefs and behavior as being extreme or unnecessary. And because avoiding meat tends to disrupt social activities—which often center around food—these individuals are strongly tempted to eat flesh now and then to fit in with their friends and family. Once people give in to this temptation, it is not long before the vegetarian diet is abandoned completely. Sharon, a former health vegetarian, described this pattern:

> I had been vegetarian for two years before I moved to San Diego. When I first arrived, I lived with two girls who ate meat and I became surrounded a lot more by fast foods. I wasn't around people advocating vegetarian diets anymore. And one of the girls I was living with was a real partier. She would invite people over and have big meals. Sometimes I would get caught up in it and lose sight of what I wanted for myself nutritionally. There would be meat in the fridge, and someone would make a bacon, lettuce, and tomato sandwich and say, "Would you like one?" So it was very easy to get a taste for meat again. During that time I kept saying to myself, "Why am I doing this?" But I was studying hard and working, and it was just inconvenient to find a new social circle.

A variation on this theme occurs among people who make the transition to vegetarianism with a partner. When the partner starts to eat meat again, the other falls off the wagon as well. As one woman said, "I tried not eating meat about 12 years ago. My boyfriend joined me at first. But he didn't last too long and began sneaking food from McDonald's. Eventually, I gave up, too."

A further variation on this theme occurs among young people still living at home whose parents are not supportive. Although children or adolescents are often able to maintain a vegetarian diet for several months, or even years, in spite of parental disapproval, most eventually give in to pressure.

> I made a declaration at 14 that I was going to be vegetarian. My family just went berserk. That lasted about two months. It was summer with lots of fruits and vegetables, so it was OK. But the family put a lot of pressure on me to eat meat, so I started again.

For many young would-be vegetarians living at home with parents, the setback is temporary; many patiently wait until they move out and then try again.

The fact that many individuals revert to flesh-eating because of a lack of social support is notable. As we described earlier, many people reach the decision to stop eating meat on their own, either through reading books or other literature, seeing films, or having "meat insight" experiences. It is not uncommon for people who reach their decisions individually to have no vegetarian friends or acquaintances. Many, in fact, have never met another vegetarian—at least, as far as they are aware. These people, if they remain socially isolated, have difficulty completing the transition successfully.

Why? A good deal of psychological research shows that people have a difficult time maintaining their beliefs and attitudes in the absence of support from others. For one thing, people do not like to feel that they are alone with their beliefs, no matter how committed they are. And people need to be rewarded now and then for acting out their beliefs; yet nonvegetarian friends and family are unlikely to offer praise or encouragement. In addition, ethical vegetarians may become discouraged and see their efforts as futile because they believe too few people are behaving similarly.

Consequently, individuals in these circumstances should make an effort to meet other vegetarians as early as possible. Many large cities have vegetarian organizations and clubs that plan social activities, and these are important but often underutilized resources. Even if there are no clubs locally, people can subscribe to newsletters and vegetarian magazines; although not as good as vegetarians "in person," they serve as reminders that others share the same beliefs and practices. And, of course, people who find no vegetarian clubs in their area can always start their own. Surveys show that between 3 and 4 percent of the United States population is vegetarian. This means that in a city with 20,000 people, there will be about 600 to 800 vegetarians. Ironically, many of these individuals probably wish they could meet other vegetarians. All it takes is for one person to organize the time and place.

Inadequate Preparation

A lack of preparation is a second major reason for abandoning vegetarianism. People who encounter this problem typically make the decision to become vegetarian quickly. However, because they are used to basic meals consisting of meat, potatoes, and a vegetable, and because they have done no preliminary reading or cooking, they literally don't know what to cook to replace the meat that is no longer on their plates. To complicate matters, these people tend to be busy with jobs and other commitments that leave little time for learning new recipes or styles of cooking. As a result, they eat bland meals consisting of simple salads, soggy vegetables, and sandwiches. Not surprisingly, as time passes, vegetarian food comes to seem increasingly dreary and meat increasingly tempting. After a while, out of a desire for convenience and a tasty meal, these people revert back to eating flesh. Lorna, a marriage counsellor, described this pattern:

> We tried to give up meat, but it was hard to plan meals without the meat course. I'd sit down with cookbooks and it would take hours to make my weekly menu and food shopping list. We were both working full-time jobs and it took too much energy to come home and cook something we'd never made before. And whole grains and legumes took so long to cook. We drifted back into eating meat again because it was so much easier, and we really liked meat.

Mike, a self-employed businessperson, experienced the same problem:

> I was vegetarian for a couple of years, but I didn't really have a well-planned diet. I hadn't educated myself. I didn't really know that much. I started to feel that I was missing out on something from my diet, and I wasn't taking the time to prepare things properly. I was just eating peanut butter sandwiches. Eventually I began to break down. I felt that I was starving, so I'd have some chicken or fish. I felt like I needed to do it.

A few people claim they became ill or that their health deteriorated after they became vegetarians. Like the people noted above, these people generally had poor-quality diets. Mary, a homemaker, made the following comments:

> I became a vegetarian at 16 and stayed that way for two years. It was difficult because I lived in a family of meat-eaters and I knew very little about nutrition. I was pretty much eating the same white flour, white sugar diet, minus the meat. As a result of my poor diet, I was thin, pale, and often ill. I went back to meat-eating in college because I figured it was the best way to improve my health.

People who are contemplating a vegetarian diet would do well to spend some time in preparation. A reasonable goal would be to learn one or two new vegetarian recipes a week. (A good vegetarian cookbook is essential for this purpose.) This initial period of learning can be brief; most people probably have a repertoire of half a dozen good recipes they regularly rely on for main meals, so an initial core of vegetarian recipes is not difficult to assemble. Contrary to popular opinion, many vegetarian dishes are quick and easy to prepare, and the novice would be better off learning these rather than gourmet dishes that take hours to cook.

When learning new recipes, we recommend that people not replace former meat dishes with recipes that rely heavily on cheese or eggs as "meat replacements." For one thing, cheese and eggs are high in cholesterol and fat, and increasing one's consumption of these products can negate some of the potential health benefits of a vegetarian diet. Second, ethical vegetarians are not completely off the hook just because they don't eat meat, for the dairy and egg industries are among the worst of all abusers of farm animals. So increasing the demand for dairy products and eggs negates much of the moral good that one accomplishes by decreasing the demand for animal flesh. Third, many lacto-ovo-vegetarians eventually decide to become vegan, or at least to minimize their consumption of eggs and dairy products. Many have a difficult time making the transition to veganism because they learned to rely heavily on dairy products during their lacto-ovo years. For them, it is like giving up meat all over again. The solution to all three problems is to replace the meat in your diet with foods of plant origin, including legumes, vegetables, grain dishes, and soy products.

Because a little preparation eases the transition considerably, we recommend that people not eliminate meat during a particularly busy or stressful period. Becoming vegetarian should be an enjoyable and exciting experience; it should not be something that contributes more stress to an already busy workday. During the initial weeks, people should have enough free time to read about vegetarian nutrition and philosophy. They should also seek out new places to shop—natural groceries, health food stores, or food cooperatives—and have a look at the variety of vegetarian foods available there. And they should try out new recipes using new foods and flavorings. Making the change should be a self-indulgent experience. A vacation, or some other nonstressful period, is a good time to get the ball rolling.

Giving in to Cravings

A third reason for ceasing to be vegetarian involves giving in to a sudden craving for meat. Although it is common for new vegetarians to have cravings for meat (and occasionally to eat meat), people who have been vegetarian for years are also susceptible. When meat is eaten impulsively, it can lead individuals to reevaluate their commitment to vegetarianism. Some feel they must not be "real vegetarians," because real vegetarians would never have succumbed to temptation. Because of the initial doubt that is raised, it is easier to give in to the next impulse—and the next. Like a small hole in a dam, the single incident eventually leads to the destruction of the vegetarian lifestyle. The following comments, one by a primary school teacher and the other by a university professor, are typical:

> For two and one half years I went really strong. Then one day I got a craving for a hamburger. I thought to myself, "That's gross. Why do I want a hamburger?" I had been eating soyburgers, but I thought, "What the heck." I went for the hamburger, and that's what broke it all. That was the beginning of the end.

> I had been vegetarian for about two years. Then I went through a period of life when I was under a great deal of stress. I lost my appetite and wasn't eating anything for a while. One day a corned beef sandwich sounded good, so I ate it. After that, I started eating meat again. I just didn't feel like a vegetarian anymore.

Our research shows that it is not uncommon for vegetarians to try meat again long after they have "stopped" eating it. But this simple act sometimes leads people to question their self-definitions as vegetarians. Because thinking of oneself as a vegetarian is an important source of motivation to remain on a meatless diet, a change in self-evaluation can serve as the first step in a process that eventually leads to the abandoning of the behavior.

A clear parallel to this phenomenon exists in the psychological literature on smoking and alcoholism, where the event is referred to as a "single relapse episode." Such an incident is typically interpreted by the individual as an inability to control a previous addiction. Often people who have successfully abstained from smoking or drinking for months or even years will give in and return to their previous addiction after a single relapse. To prevent this, psychologists prepare their clients for situations where this might occur by helping them to realize that giving in to temptation on a single occasion is common; it does not mean that they are failures or that they are incapable of further self-control. Vegetarians should adopt a similar attitude.

In the case of abstaining from meat, a relapse often results in a change in self-concept because many people—vegetarians and meat-eaters—hold an overly rigid notion of what it means to be a vegetarian. They believe that a "true" vegetarian must be 100 percent consistent and completely pure in beliefs and behavior. According to this view, a single relapse means that a person is no longer a vegetarian. But it makes more sense to describe people by their typical rather than atypical behavior. Consequently, when vegetarians give in to a sudden craving or impulse to eat a hot dog or a piece of chicken, they should think of themselves as vegetarians who slipped up—but as vegetarians nonetheless. They should *not* see themselves as failures just because they engage in a behavior that is temporarily "out of role."

A Weak Commitment

Finally, some people stop being vegetarian because they are not strongly committed in the first place. Sometimes these individuals try a meatless diet because they are curious to find out what it feels like. In other cases they do it to fit in better with family or friends who are vegetarians. Their lack of commitment, however, means that the experiment is typically short-lived. Nevertheless, although these attempts are unsuccessful, they sometimes set the stage for later, more serious, commitments to vegetarianism. Rhonda, a secretary, told us about her earlier attempts to give up meat and how they differed from her current situation:

> I had made several attempts in the past 20 years to become vegetarian but without much success beyond about three months. The reason I have been successful this time, I believe, is because in the past I did not have the moral conviction that I now have to sustain my efforts. My motives for becoming vegetarian then were for health reasons and vaguely for humanitarian reasons.

As we pointed out earlier, if you want to remain vegetarian, you should be clear about your motives. Of course, it is fine to experiment with vegetarianism, even if you have put little thought into it. After all, there is nothing to lose, and you might discover that you like it. But the more seriously you approach your decision, the more you will get out of the experience in the long run.

THE FUTURE OF VEGETARIANISM

When a group is small in size, its impact on the larger society is minimal; but as it grows, its influence becomes inevitable. Indeed, at this point in time, a "critical mass" of vegetarians can be said to exist, and they have already begun to leave their mark on our society. Presently, vegetarians are numerous enough to provide markets for vegetarian magazines, books, food products, restaurants, clothing, cosmetics, personal care products, and other goods. In addition, stereotypes are beginning to change; compared with previous times, people today are less likely to see vegetarians as extreme or fanatical and are more likely to see them as normal and sensible.

As time goes on, the number of vegetarians in our society will undoubtedly increase. How far will this trend go? In principle, vegetarianism is attainable by everyone; it is not necessary for anyone to eat animal flesh. Of course, it is unlikely that the majority of people in the West will become strict vegetarians in the next few years. Nevertheless, a change in dietary habits is already occurring within the broad majority. It is not difficult to imagine that in 50 years' time, most people will be semivegetarians, eating meat occasionally, but living primarily on plant foods.

What will be the implications of such a change? Some might think that what we eat, in the larger scheme of things, is not very important. But eating is an activity that we engage in several times every day. And the choice of what we eat is bound up with our health, the economy, the environment, and our philosophy of life. In our opinion, the beneficial impact of a large-scale shift to vegetarianism, or even semivegetarianism, will be profound.

In terms of health, medical studies indicate that it is possible to lower serum cholesterol levels by switching to a low-fat, low-cholesterol, high-fiber diet.[1] This is accompanied by a decrease—and even a reversal—in the buildup of plaque on artery walls. The overall effect of these changes is a decrease in the likelihood of contracting coronary heart disease. Presently, coronary heart disease is the leading killer in the United States. Any measure that helps to bring it under control will have major implications for public health.

Readers may be interested to know that during the last 20 years, mortality rates from coronary heart disease have been declining in the United States. In fact, between the early 1960s and the early 1980s, mortality rates dropped by 37 percent. Why has this decline occurred? A recent study compared the impact of several factors on this change: improvements in five medical treatments (including coronary artery bypass surgery and drug therapy), reduction in fat consumption, and reduction in cigarette smoking. As it turned out, medical treatments were estimated to be responsible for about 40 percent of the decline in mortality rates, whereas the two lifestyle changes accounted for over half of the decline. In particular, cholesterol reduction was estimated to account for about 30 percent of the decline, with the reduction in smoking accounting for a further 24 percent.[2]

These figures indicate that simple lifestyle changes—changes that are under the direct control of individuals—have greater implications for the reduction of heart disease than do complex and expensive medical procedures. Translated into lives, the reduction in cholesterol consumption in the United States during the last 20 years has resulted in 150,000 fewer deaths than would otherwise have been expected. Clearly, prevention, rather than reliance on medical technology, is the best strategy for dealing with this major public health problem.

Although these figures are impressive, they are only a hint of what is possible. The reduction in cholesterol consumption in the United States, when all is said and done, has been minimal; although many people are eating less beef and eggs than they used to, the diet of the average American continues to be largely based on animal products. Anyone who doubts this can examine the dinner menus of virtually any restaurant in the country—excluding vegetarian restaurants, of course—and count the number of main courses not based on meat or fish. People who carry out this investigation will discover that there are few, if any. And if there is a fleshless dish on the menu, it will no doubt include eggs (which are high in cholesterol) or be smothered in cheese (which is high in fat). Without doubt, a large-scale adoption of a low-fat, low-cholesterol, high-fiber diet based mainly on plant foods will lead to a more dramatic decline in the rate of heart disease mortality than we have presently seen.

In addition, as we pointed out earlier, rates of several forms of cancer, including cancer of the colon and breast, are correlated with fat consumption. Given that over one third of cancer deaths can be attributed to what we eat,[3] the adoption of a vegetarian or semivegetarian diet that includes generous servings of fruits, vegetables, legumes, and whole grain products will be a major step in bringing current rates of cancer under control.

In addition to coronary heart disease and cancer, which are devastating health problems in the West, the widespread adoption of vegetarianism will have implications for the daily quality of life. Eating a nutritionally balanced diet is an important health-promoting behavior. And although "junk food" vegetarians are not unknown, the majority of vegetarians—regardless of their motives for not eating meat—have been attracted to unprocessed whole foods. Fresh fruits and vegetables, as well as whole grain products, can be found in abundance in the homes of most vegetarians. In addition, keeping physically active has been part of the traditional vegetarian lifestyle. People who eat well and keep fit not only avoid illness—they also feel good and look good. Vegetarianism, as part of a larger package of behaviors aimed at maintaining optimal health, will ensure that the daily well-being of people in our society is maximized.

In terms of the environment, we noted that livestock production bears much of the responsibility for our present ecological problems. Massive deforestation, desertification, soil erosion, and water pollution are the prices we have paid to have meat on our plates every night. Yet, as the demand for meat decreases, market forces will lead agriculturalists to turn to alternative products that are less damaging to the environment. For example, an increasing demand for organically grown produce (fruits and vegetables grown without pesticides) suggests a new market for agriculturalists to satisfy. (Pesticides do a good deal of harm to wildlife, so an increase in the production of organically grown crops would result in less stress being placed on the ecology.)

Of course, it is possible to feed more people per acre by growing plant foods than by producing animal foods, so less land will be required to meet food needs in a semivegetarian society. This means that much of the land presently used for cattle grazing or for the growing of cattle feed can be used for other purposes. Some of this land, left undisturbed, will eventually return to woodlands and can be used as a future source of timber. Other land can be converted into nature reserves.

Given the number of animal and plant species currently under threat of extinction, the setting aside of additional land for nature reserves is imperative. This land will need to be unfenced to allow the natural migration of animals in times of unusual weather, such as drought or cold, and to minimize inbreeding of local populations. Currently, most privately owned land, as well as large areas of present nature reserves, are fenced to allow cattle grazing. (And as we noted earlier, present cattle grazing poses a long-term risk to our parks and reserves due to its effects on soil erosion.) The creation of additional reserves, unfenced and free of dense herds of grazing cattle, will help to stem the rapid loss of our irreplaceable wildlife.

Will a move away from a meat-centered diet lead to massive economic disruption for agriculturalists? It is true that fewer people will need to be employed in agricultural industries in a vegetarian economy. The meat industry, in particular, will have seen better days. However, massive disruption seems unlikely, given that society-wide changes in behavior tend to occur gradually. Some disruption is probably inevitable, but this is a fact of life in a competitive economy. Indeed, because of changes in technology, the proportion of people employed in agriculture has decreased steadily during the last century. In this light, vegetarianism can be seen as simply one more step in making agricultural production more efficient.

Of course, a degree of economic disruption cannot be used as a rationale for opposing vegetarianism. Consider the antismoking movement. Clearly, the larger good is served by encouraging people to stop smoking, even though this may result in some temporary economic hardship to those employed in the tobacco and cigarette industries.

Because plant foods are less wasteful of land, water, and energy than are animal foods, they have the potential to feed a hungry world. The majority of the world's population will never live on a meat-centered diet; the earth does not have the resources to provide every person with the diet of the average American. People in the West, it seems, have been eating more than their share. Starvation can be eradicated in the Third World, given improvements in agricultural technology, a switch from cash crops that feed no one (such as rubber and coffee) to crops such as grains and legumes, and political changes that allow a redistribution of land from the rich to the poor. As the Third World develops, people there will look to the West for models to emulate; but it is irresponsible to hold up our meat-centered diet as the ideal to be pursued. The world can only be well-fed if the majority of its people live as vegetarians.

In terms of ethics, a large-scale rejection of a meat-centered diet will lead to a massive reduction in the number of animals forced to live under miserable conditions on factory farms. There is a direct correlation between consumer demand for meat and the number of animals bred for slaughter. If consumer demand decreases, market forces will depress the price of meat, and, correspondingly, agriculturalists will reduce the supply by breeding fewer animals for slaughter. Ethical vegetarians look forward to the day when factory farms will be totally eradicated. In the meantime, they see every decrease in the amount of suffering experienced by animals as a small moral victory.

Finally, we might consider the effects of widespread vegetarianism on the mental health of the population. We found earlier that vegetarians experience increments in energy level, self-esteem, perceptions of control, feelings of peacefulness, and sense of moral purpose in life. Perhaps the adoption of vegetarianism on a society-wide level would lead to a general improvement in the psychological well-being of the population. If nothing else, encouraging our children to protect their physical health, respect all forms of life, live nonviolently, and care about the quality of the natural environment—values that are part and parcel of vegetarianism—would ensure that future generations adopt a sensitive and responsible attitude toward the world and their place in it. These future generations might be more successful than we have been in finding solutions to pressing problems, such as achieving world peace and learning how to live in harmony with nature.

Given these benefits, we think it likely that the majority of people in the West will one day live as vegetarians. In the meantime, a low-fat, high-fiber diet centered on plant foods, supplemented with occasional small servings of animal protein, is a practical and achievable goal for most people. Of course, it is also the diet eaten by our early ancestors. Our modern Western diet based on meat and other animal products is an aberration—and one which has had negative consequences for our well-being.

A return to a traditional diet, however, does not imply that our meals need be limited or tedious, as they may have been during previous eras. Instead, a modern plant-based diet is enriched by the diversity and abundance of plant foods now available to us, by the sharing of ethnic cuisines from around the world, and by new products being developed by vegetarian food industries.

Vegetarianism is not a panacea for the ills of the world. But from the point of view of health, ethics, and the environment, vegetarianism represents a practical lifestyle well-suited to our own needs, and the needs of the planet, as we move into the next millenium.

People can be frustratingly slow in modifying their behavior, but they can change. We close this chapter with a quotation from Brenda, which summarizes the feelings of many vegetarians as they contemplate the future:

> Sometimes I look at all the people in cars on the highway, or at big apartment buildings, or at the people in malls, movie theaters, or stadium events, and I realize that most, if not all of them, eat meat. And I think about the number of animals they will consume that day, and the number of animals they will consume in a lifetime, and all the suffering it entails. I look at fat people, and people suffering from degenerative illness, and know that they could be thin and healthy if they adopted a vegetarian diet. And I think of all the starving people who live in countries that export meat and about how they would have enough to eat if their

governments changed their agricultural policies. And I find it incomprehensible how such a simple solution to so many problems can be overlooked by most, and violently rejected by others. Yet, I have to remind myself how long it took me to get there.

Vegetarian Resources

ORGANIZATIONS

The following organizations may be useful for people who wish to find out more about vegetarianism. Many of these organizations can provide lists of affiliated vegetarian groups and contacts for those who wish to join a local group. Many also publish newsletters and sell books on vegetarianism through the mail.

The American Vegan Society
Box H (Old Harding Highway)
Malaga, NJ 08328

Animal Liberation
20 Enmore Road
Newtown, NSW 2042
Australia

Baltimore Vegetarians
P.O. Box 1463
Baltimore, MD 21203

Farm Animal Reform Movement
P.O. Box 70123
Washington, DC 20088

International Vegetarian Union
10 Kings Drive
Marple
Stockport, Cheshire SK6 6NQ
England

New Zealand Vegetarian Society
P.O. Box 454
Auckland 1
New Zealand

North American Vegetarian Society
P.O. Box 72
Dolgeville, NY 13329

Toronto Vegetarian Association
28 Walker Avenue
Toronto ON M4V 1G2
Canada

Association of Vegetarian Dietitians and Nutrition Educators (VEGEDINE)
1225 Lenox Avenue
Miami, FL 33139

(VEGEDINE publishes *Issues in Vegetarian Dietetics*. Contact VEGEDINE for the name and address of the nearest vegetarian registered dietician.)

The Vegetarian Union of North America
P.O. Box 9710
Washington, DC 20016

The Vegan Society
33-35 George Street
Oxford OX1 2AY
England

The Vegan Society of Australia
P.O. Box 85
Seaford
Victoria, 3198
Australia

MAGAZINES

The Animals' Agenda
456 Monroe Turnpike
Monroe, CT 06468

The Animals' Agenda is useful reading for those interested in the treatment of animals and environmental issues.

Vegetarian Times
P.O. Box 570
Oak Park, IL 60303

Vegetarian Times is a monthly magazine that covers a range of vegetarian issues. Its special-issue publication, "The Essential Guide to Dining, Leisure, Clubs and Products" is recommended. It provides a comprehensive listing of restaurants and organizations in the United States of interest to vegetarians.

BOOKS

The following books are useful resources for readers who wish to explore some possible ingredients of a vegetarian lifestyle.

Cookbooks

Laurel Robertson, *The New Laurel's Kitchen* (Berkeley, CA: Ten Speed Press, 1986).

Frank J. Hurd and Rosalie Hurd, *Ten Talents* (Collegedale, TN: Collegedale Press, 1985).
The Cookbook for People Who Love Animals (Umatilla, FL: Gentle World, 1985).

Nutrition

Jane Brody, *Jane Brody's Nutrition Book* (NY: Bantam, 1987).
John A. McDougall and Mary A. McDougall, *The McDougall Plan* (Piscataway, NJ: New Century, 1983).

Interested readers might also wish to look up Suzanne Havala and Johanna Dwyer, "Position of the American Dietetic Association: Vegetarian Diets," *Journal of the American Dietetic Association* 88 (March 1988), pp. 352–353, for an authoritative and nontechnical statement on vegetarian nutrition.

References

Chapter 1

1. Joel Gurin, "Are You a Semi-Vegetarian?" *American Health* (July/August 1985), pp. 37–43.
2. "Dining Out Becomes Healthier," *Vegetarian Times* (February 1986), p. 7.
3. "The Essential Guide to Dining, Leisure, Clubs, Products," *Vegetarian Times* (July 1987), pp. 27–75.
4. Ron Givens, "Going for the Greens," *Newsweek* (May 9, 1986), pp. 79–80.
5. Sheila Gribben and Andrea Sachs, "Vegetarians Hit the Fern Bars," *Time* (March 7, 1988), p. 84.
6. Gretel H. Pelto and Pertti, J. Pelto, *The Human Adventure* (New York: Macmillan, 1976), pp. 203–204.
7. Discussions of the history of vegetarianism can be found in: Keith Akers, *A Vegetarian Sourcebook* (Arlington, VA: Vegetarian Press, 1983), pp. 180–187; Daniel A. Dombrowski, *The Philosophy of Vegetarianism* (Amherst: The University of Massachusetts Press, 1984); Dudley Giehl, *Vegetarianism: A Way of Life* (New York: Harper and Row, 1979); James Turner, *Reckoning with the Beast: Animals, Pain, and Humanity in the Victorian Mind* (Baltimore: The Johns Hopkins University Press, 1980); "Vegetarianism," *Encyclopaedia Brittanica* 22 (Chicago: William Bentor, 1969), pp. 935–945.
8. Leonardo da Vinci's notebook, quoted in Victoria Moran, "Leonardo da Vinci: A Portrait of a Renaissance Man," *Vegetarian Times* (October 1987) pp. 23–26.
9. Some recent examples include: M. Abdulla *et al.*, "Nutritional Intake and Health Status of Lacto-ovo Vegetarians," *American Journal of Clinical Nutrition* 40 (1984), pp. 325–338; Beverly Calkins, D. J. Whittaker, A. A. Rider, and N. Turjman, "Nutritional Intake," *American Journal of Clinical Nutrition* 40 (1984), pp. 896–905; E. Carlson, M. Kipps, A. Lockie, and J. Thomas, "A Comparative Evaluation of Vegan, Vegetarian, and Omnivore Diets," *Journal of Plant Foods* 6 (1985), pp. 89–100; A. Rider, R. S. Arthur, B. M. Calkins, and P. Nair, "Selected Biochemical Parameters in Blood and Urine," *American Journal of Clinical Nutrition* 40 (1984), pp. 917–920.
10. "Vegetarianism: Can You Get By Without Meat?" *Consumer Reports* (June 1980), pp. 357–365.

11. Suzanne Havala and Johanna Dwyer, "Position of the American Dietetic Association: Vegetarian Diets—Technical Support Paper," *Journal of the American Dietetic Association* 88 (March 1988), p. 352.
12. National Research Council, *Recommended Dietary Allowances* (Washington, D.C.: National Academy of Sciences, 1980).
13. Havala, p. 353; John A. McDougall and Mary A. McDougall, *The McDougall Plan* (Piscataway, NJ: New Century, 1983), Chapter 8.
14. U.S. Department of Agriculture, *Nutritive Value of American Foods*, Agriculture Handbook No. 456 (Washington, D.C.: U.S. Government Printing Office, 1975).
15. Havala, p. 353.
16. Frances Moore Lappé, *Diet for a Small Planet: Tenth Anniversary Edition* (New York: Ballantine, 1982).
17. Peter Burwash and John Tallias, *Peter Burwash's Vegetarian Primer* (New York: Atheneum, 1983); John Robbins, *Diet for a New America* (Walpole, NH: Stillpoint, 1987), pp. 155–163.
18. Janie C. Hartbarger and Neil J. Hartbarger, *Eating for the Eighties: A Complete Guide to Vegetarian Nutrition* (Philadelphia: W. B. Saunders, 1980).
19. Catherine Saxelby, *Nutrition for Life* (French's Forest, Victoria, Australia: Reed Books), pp. 62–63; McDougall, pp. 132–143.
20. George Eisman, "Vegetarians and Vitamin D," *Vegetarian Voice* 12 (1986).
21. S. J. Baker, "Human Vitamin B-12 Deficiency," *World Review of Nutrition and Dietetics* 8 (1967), pp. 62–126; A. D. M. Smith, "Veganism, A Clinical Survey with Observations of Vitamin B-12 Metabolism," *The British Medical Journal* 1 (June 1962), p. 1655.
22. Richard Bargen, *The Vegetarian's Self-Defense Manual* (Wheaton, IL: Quest Books), p. 97.
23. Akers, p. 37; Michael Klapper, *Vegan Nutrition* (Umatilla, FL: Gentle World, 1988).
24. "Contribution of the Microflora of the Small Intestine to the Vitamin B-12 Nutriture of Man," *Nutrition Reviews* 38 (1980), pp. 274–275; M. Albert, "Vitamin B12 Synthesis by Human Small Intestinal Bacteria," *Nature* 283 (1981), p. 2423.
25. Abdulla, pp. 325–338; A. H. Lockie, E. Carlson, M. Kipps, and J. Thomas, "Comparison of Four Types of Diet Using Clinical, Laboratory, and Psychological Studies," *Journal of the Royal College of General Practitioners* 35 (1985), pp. 333–336.
26. J. Stamler, "Population Studies," in R. I. Levy, B. M. Rifkind, B. H. Dennis, and N. Ernst (Eds.), *Nutrition, Lipids, and Coronary Heart Disease* (New York: Raven Press, 1979).
27. Leslie Goodman-Malamuth, "McHeartbreak: Cardiologists Underscore Danger of a High-Fat Diet at Fast-Food Restaurants," *Nutrition Action Health Letter*, Center for Science in the Public Interest (January 1986), pp. 10–11.
28. *The American Heart Association Diet* (Dallas: The American Heart Association, 1985).

29. Havala, p. 352.
30. M. L. Burr and P. M. Sweetnam, "Vegetarianism, Dietary Fiber, and Mortality," *American Journal of Clinical Nutrition* 36 (1982), p. 873; R. L. Phillips *et al.*, "Coronary Heart Disease Mortality among Seventh-Day Adventists with Differing Dietary Habits: A Preliminary Report," *American Journal of Clinical Nutrition* 31 (1978), p. 191; R. L. Phillips, J. W. Kuzma, W. L. Beeson, and T. Lotz, "Influence of Selection Versus Lifestyle on Risk of Fatal Cancer and Cardio-vascular Disease Among Seventh-Day Adventists," *American Journal of Epidemiology* 112 (1980), p. 296.
31. John W. Berg, William Haenszel, and Susan S. Devesa, "Epidemiology of Gastrointestinal Cancer," *Proceedings of the Seventh National Cancer Conference*, American Cancer Society and the National Cancer Institute (Philadelphia: J. B. Lippincott, 1972), p. 459; Daniel G. Miller, "Cancer Prevention: Steps You Can Take," in Arthur Holleb (Ed.), *The American Cancer Society Cancer Book* (New York: Doubleday, 1986), pp. 15–40; E. Wynder, "The Dietary Environment and Cancer," *Journal of the American Dietetic Association* 71 (1977), p. 385.
32. Lorelei DiSogra, and Charles DiSogra, *Diet, Nutrition, and Cancer Prevention: A Guide to Food Choices*, NIH Publication No. 85-2711 (Washington, D.C.: U.S. Department of Health and Human Services, 1984), p. 5.
33. *Ibid.*
34. *Nutrition and Cancer: Cause and Prevention* (American Cancer Society, undated brochure).
35. Information on the link between diet and cancer can be found in articles in the following sources: Jerome J. DeCosse, "Cancer of the Colon and Rectum," in Arthur I. Holleb (Ed.), *The American Cancer Society Cancer Book* (New York: Doubleday, 1986), pp. 341–361; Bandura S. Reddy and Leonard Cohen (Eds.), *Diet, Nutrition, and Cancer: A Critical Evaluation. Volume 1. Macronutrients and Cancer* (Boca Raton: CRC Press, 1986); Bandura S. Reddy and Leonard Cohen (Eds.), *Diet, Nutrition, and Cancer: A Critical Evaluation. Volume 2. Micronutrients and Cancer* (Boca Raton: CRC Press, 1986), Myron Winick (Ed.), *Nutrition and Cancer* (New York: Wiley, 1977).
36. *Facts You Should Know about Outdoor Cooking* (Washington, D.C.: American Institute for Cancer Research, 1986).
37. Akers, pp. 65–74; Havala, pp. 352–353; R. L. Phillips, L. Garfinkel, J. W. Kuzma, W. L. Beeson, T. Lotz, and B. Brin, "Mortality among California Seventh-Day Adventists for Selected Cancer Sites," *Journal of the National Cancer Institute* 65 (1980), p. 1097; Robbins, pp. 248–273.
38. Akers, pp. 75–80; Havala, p. 353; Robbins, pp. 274–305.
39. Greg Moyer, "Osteoporosis: The Disease," Nutrition Action Newsletter (Washington, D.C.: Center for Science in the Public Interest, 1985), pp. 4–9, 14; Carol M. Cain, "The Calcium Hoopla: Are You Being Misled?" *Vegetarian Times* (May 1987), pp. 47–49, 67.
40. Penny W. Moser, "It Must Have Been Something You Ate," *Discover* (February 1987), pp. 94–100.

41. R. H. Kahn, R. L. Philips, D. A. Snowdon, and W. Choi, "Association Between Reported Diet and All Cause Mortality: Twenty-one Year Follow Up on 27,530 Seventh-Day Adventists," *American Journal of Epidemiology* 119 (1984), p. 775.
42. Sources for this section include Akers, pp. 169–179; Louis A. Berman, *Vegetarianism and the Jewish Tradition,* (New York: KTAV Publishing House, 1982); John Cook, *Diet and Your Religion* (Santa Barbara: Woodridge Press, 1976); International Society for Krishna Consciousness, *The Higher Taste* (New York: Bhaktivedanta Books, 1983); Philip Kepleau, *To Cherish All Life: A Buddhist Case for Becoming Vegetarian* (San Francisco: Harper and Row, 1981); Phillip L. Pick (Ed.), *Tree of Life: An Anthology of Articles Appearing in the Jewish Vegetarian* (Cranbury, NJ: A. S. Barnes, 1977).
43. Lappé, 1982, pp. 66–74.
44. *Ibid.*, p. 66.
45. Lappé, 1982, pp. 76–79; Akers, pp. 101–111.
46. Lappé, 1982, pp. 79–83; Akers, pp. 117–121.
47. Lynn Jacobs, "Amazing Grace: How the Livestock Industry Is Ruining the American West," *The Animals' Agenda* (January 1988), pp. 12–17.
48. Lappé, 1982, p. 84.
49. Frances Moore Lappé, *Food First: Beyond the Myth of Scarcity* (New York: Ballantine Books, 1978), pp. 84–53.
50. Lappé, 1982, p. 69.
51. Gordon Gallup, "Our Use and/or Abuse of Animals: Is Research a Special Case?," paper presented at the Western Psychological Association 67th Annual Convention, Long Beach, California, April 23–26, 1987.
52. Discussions of factory farming methods and conditions can be found in Michael W. Fox, *Farm Animals: Husbandry, Behavior, and Veterinary Practice* (Baltimore: University Park Press, 1983); Bradley S. Miller, "The Violence in the Egg Carton," *The Animals' Agenda* (September 1987), pp. 28–32, 57; Jim Mason and Peter Singer, *Animal Factories* (New York: Crown Publishers, 1980); Robbins, pp. 48–145; Peter Singer, *Animal Liberation* (New York: Avon Books, 1975).
53. Singer, 1975.
54. Tom Regan, *The Case for Animal Rights* (Berkeley: University of California Press, 1983).
55. Bryan Kolb and Ian Q. Whishaw, *Fundamentals of Human Neuro-psychology* (San Francisco, W. H. Freeman, 1980), pp. 89–107.
56. Ronald Melzack, "The Perception of Pain," *Science* (February 1961), pp. 223–231.
57. Kolb and Whishaw, p. 89.
58. Dallas Pratt, *Alternatives to Pain in Experiments on Animals* (New York: Argus Archives, 1980), pp. 11–30.
59. F. J. J. Buytendijk, *Pain* (Westport, CT: Greenwood Press, 1973), pp. 71–106.
60. Jane van Lawick-Goodall, *In the Shadow of Man* (New York: Dell Publishing, 1971).

61. Steven Green and Peter Marler, "The Analysis of Animal Communications," in Peter Marler and J. G. Vandenbergh (Eds.), *Handbook of Behavioral Neurobiology. Volume 3. Social Behavior and Communication* (New York: Plenum, 1979), pp. 73–158.
62. John Alcock, *Animal Behavior* (Sunderland, MA: Sinauer Associates, 1984), pp. 467–504.
63. *Ibid.*
64. R. Allen Gardner and T. Beatrice, "Teaching Sign Language to a Chimpanzee," *Science* 165 (1975), pp. 664–672.
65. M. Ray Denny, "Complex Behavior," in M. Ray Denny (Ed.), *Comparative Psychology* (New York: Wiley, 1980), pp. 249–266.
66. Mohandas Gandhi, *The Story of My Experiments with Truth* (New York: Beacon Press, 1957).
67. Porphry, cited in Kepleau, p. 34.
68. Kepleau, p. 55.
69. Isaac Bashevis Singer, "Foreword," in Giehl, p. ix.
70. Henry David Thoreau, *Walden* (Princeton, NJ: Princeton University Press, 1971), pp. 214–215.

Chapter 4

1. "How Do You Feel?" *Vegetarian Times* (November 1987), p. 14.
2. Suzanne Havala and Johanna Dwyer, "Position of the American Dietetic Association: Vegetarian Diets—Technical Support Paper," *Journal of the American Dietetic Association* 88 (March 1988), pp. 352–355.
3. Jeanne H. Freeland-Graves, Sue A. Greninger, Glenn R. Graves, and Robert K. Young, "Health Practices, Attitudes, and Beliefs of Vegetarians and Nonvegetarians," *Journal of the American Dietetic Association* 86 (1986), pp. 913–918.
4. Lucy Mall, "The Popeye Phenomenon," *Vegetarian Times* (June 1986), pp. 24–30.
5. Judith J. Wurtman and Margaret Danbrot, *Managing Your Mind and Mood Through Food* (Boston: Interneuron, 1986).
6. John A. McDougall and Mary A. McDougall, *The McDougall Plan* (Piscataway, NJ: New Century Publishers, 1983), p. 85.
7. McDougall, 1983, Chapter 5.
8. Wurtman, 1986.
9. McDougall, 1983, Chapter 5.
10. Freeland-Graves, 1986./bb

Chapter 5

1. Jeanne H. Freeland Graves, Sue A. Greninger, and Robert K. Young, "A Demographic and Social Profile of Age- and Sex-Matched Vegetarians and

Nonvegetarians," *Journal of the American Dietetic Association* 86 (1986), pp. 907–913.

Chapter 6

1. Jeanne H. Freeland-Graves, Sue A. Greninger, and Robert K. Young, "A Demographic and Social Profile of Age- and Sex-Matched Vegetarians and Nonvegetarians," *Journal of the American Dietetic Association* 86 (1986), pp. 907–913.
2. *Ibid.*

Chapter 7

1. Janie C. Hartbarger and Neil J. Hartbarger, *Eating for the Eighties: A Complete Guide to Vegetarian Nutrition* (Philadelphia: W. B. Saunders, 1981); Suzanne Havala and Johanna Dwyer, "Position of the American Dietetic Association: Vegetarian Diets—Technical Support Paper," *Journal of the American Dietetic Association* 88 (March 1988), p. 352; Michael Klapper, *Pregnancy, Children, and the Vegan Diet* (Umatilla, FL: Gentle World, 1988); I. B. Vyhmeister, U. D. Register, and L. M. Sonnenberg, "Safe Vegetarian Diets for Children," *Pediatric Clinics of North America* 24 (1985), pp. 203–210.
2. Hartbarger, 1981.
3. "How Are the Kids?," *Vegetarian Times* (March 1988), p. 14.
4. "It Takes the Cake," *Vegetarian Times* (June 1987), p. 13.

Chapter 8

1. Eugene R. Passamani, "Cholesterol Reduction in Coronary Artery Bypass Patients," *Journal of the American Medical Association* (June 1987), pp. 3721–3722.
2. "The Good News About Heart Attacks," *University of California, Berkeley Wellness Newsletter* (May 1985), p. 1; L. Goldman and E. F. Cook, "The Decline in Ischemic Heart Disease Mortality Rates," *Annals of Internal Medicine* 101 (1984), pp. 825–836; J. Stamler, "Primary Prevention of Coronary Heart Disease: The Last 20 Years," *American Journal of Cardiology* 47 (1984), pp. 722–735.
3. Lorelei DiSogra and Charles DiSogra, *Diet, Nutrition, and Cancer Prevention: A Guide to Food Choices*, NIH Publication No. 85-2711 (Washington, D.C.: U.S. Department of Health and Human Services, 1984), p. 5.

Index

Aesthetics, 44–45
Age, 33, 112–113
Aggression, 118–119
Alcohol, 149–150, 258
American Dietetic Association, 6, 7–8, 104
American Heart Association, 11
American Institute for Cancer Research, 13
Amino acids, 7–8
Anger, 123, 125–126
Animal rights, 21–27
  leather products, 151–153
  motivation, 35–38
  pets, 162
  psychological factors, 119, 120, 123–126
  sex role, 219
  social relations, 189
  transition period, 68, 70–77, 78–79
  vegetarian future, 264
Anorexia nervosa, 245
Aquinas, Saint Thomas, 3
Augustine, Saint, 3

Barbecued foods, 13
Bargen, Richard, 9
Benzopyrene, 13
Biology dissection, 76
Books
  listing of, 268–269
  transition period, 68–70
Buddhism, 16–17
Bulimia, 245

Calcium, 8, 222
Cancer, 12–13, 104, 261–262
Carbohydrates, 121–122
Carcinogens, 13
Cattle production, *see* Livestock production
Cheese, 142–143
Child rearing, 222–238
  diets, 225–226
  explaining vegetarianism, 227–229
  health concerns, 222–225
  long-term prospects, 237–238
  problem avoidance, 235–237
  problems in, 232–235
  strictness, 229–232
Children
  nutrition, 8
  slaughter of animals, 74–75
Cholesterol
  heart disease, 11
  nutrition, 10
  vegetarian future, 260, 261
Christianity, 17–18
Cigarette smoking, 149–150, 258, 261, 263
Colds, 107–108
Colon cancer, 12–13
Compassion, 121
Complexion, 111

Conservationism, *see* Environmentalism
Constipation, 110–111
Cookbooks, 268–269
Coronary heart disease, 10–12, 104, 260–261
Cowherd, William, 4
Cravings, 88–91, 257–259

Dairy products, 98–99
Darwin, Charles, 3–4
Dating, 205–211; *see also* Intimate relationships; Social relations
Da Vinci, Leonardo, 3
Desertification, 19–20
Diabetes, 104
Diet
  children, 225–226
  health and, v
  nutrition and, 6–10
  see also Nutrition
Dissections, 76
Divorce, 216–218
Drugs, 149–150

Eating disorders, 245
Economic motivation, 51
Eggs, 98–99
Employment, 168–173
Energy levels, 105–107
Environmentalism
  future, 262–264
  motivation, 49–50
  vegetarianism and, 18–21
Erosion, 19
Ethics, *see* Animal rights
Evolution, 3–4, 25–26

Family, 175–182
  change over time, 180–182
  child rearing, 222–238
  conflict avoidance, 246–250
  extended visits with, 197–199
  initial reactions of, 176–180
  psychological factors, 123–124
Family (*cont.*)
  transition period, 64–65
  see also Child rearing; Marriage
Farm commune, 165–166
Fasting, 148–149
Fats
  cancer, 13
  heart disease, 11
  nutrition, 10
Films, 79–81
Financial motivation, 51
Fingernails, 111
Fishing and hunting, 178
Food allergies, 109–110
  psychological factors, 119
  soy products, 139
Friends, *see* Social relations

Gandhi, Mohandas, 27
Gentle World commune, 165
Groundwater, 20
Guilt, 119–120

Hair, 111
Health, 5–15, 103–116
  cancer, 12–13
  children, 222–225
  constipation, 110–111
  coronary heart disease, 10–12
  diet and, v
  energy increases, 105–107
  family and, 176–177, 246
  hair and complexion, 111
  illness and, 107–108
  improvements in, 103–104, 113
  issues in, 14–15
  motivation, 38–40
  nutrition and, 6–10
  positive changes, 104–113
  preexisting conditions, 108–110
  problems, 113–115
  reliability of reports, 115–116
  vegetarian future, 260–262
  weight loss, 111–112
  youthfulness, 112–113

Heart disease, 10–12, 104, 260–261
Hinduism, 15–16
Home economics courses, 236
Hospitals, 167
Humanitarian reform movement, 4
Hunting and fishing, 178
Hypertension, 104

Institutions, 166–168
Intelligence, 122
International Vegetarian Union, 5
Interpersonal relationships, *see* Family; Intimate relationships; Social relations
Intimate relationships, 205–238
  child rearing, 222–238
  conflict avoidance, 246–250
  dating, 205–211
  divorce, 216–218
  mixed couples, 213–216
  sex role, 219–221
  vegetarian couples, 211–212
  see also Family; Marriage; Social relations
Iron, 8, 222
Isolation, 123–124

Judaism, 17

Kepleau, Philip, 28
Kolb, Brian, 25

Labeling (products), 141–142
Lacto-ovo-vegetarians, 33
  family response to, 176, 180
  transition period, 96, 97, 98
Lacto-vegetarians, 33, 96, 98
Lappé, Frances Moore, 7, 8, 19, 21
Lifestyle, 137–174
  alternative diets, 137–149
  communities, 165–166
  drugs, 149–150
  employment, 168–173
  fasting, 148–149
  institutions, 166–168
Lifestyle (*cont.*)
  leather products, 150–153
  organizations, 163–165
  pets, 161–163
  restaurants, 153–157
  shopping, 144–146
  travel, 157–160
  see also Intimate relationships; Social relations
Livestock production
  animal rights , 22–23
  environment, 19–21
Living arrangements, 196–197
Longevity, 14

Magazines, 268; *see also* Media
Marijuana, 150
Marriage
  conflict avoidance, 249–250
  divorce, 216–218
  mixed couples, 213–216
  vegetarian couples, 211–212
Meat, *see* Animal rights
Meat substitutes
  alternative diets, 140–141
  cravings, 89–90
Media
  listing of resources, 268–269
  transition period, 68–70, 79–81
Meditation, 77–78
Mental health, *see* Well-being
Military, 166–167
Morality, 117–118
Mormons, 43
Motivation, 31–61
  aesthetics, 44–45
  animal ethics, 35–38
  changes over time in, 54–56
  characteristics of vegetarians, 32–34
  economics, 51
  environmentalism, 49–50
  factors in, 63–64
  health, 38–40
  idiosyncratic motives, 52–53

Motivation (*cont.*)
  naturalness, 50–51
  nonviolence, 48–49
  overview of, 53–54
  personal growth, 45–46
  religion, 40–44
  social conformity, 52
  statistical breakdown of, 34–35
  variety in, 56–61
  world hunger, 47–48
  see also Transition period

National Academy of Sciences–National Research Council, 6, 7
Natural life style, 50–51
Neuropsychology, 24–25
Nonviolence, 48–49
Nutrition
  books on, 269
  children, 222–225
  future, 262
  health, 6–10, 107
  information about, 242
  meat substitutes, 89–90
  psychological changes, 121–122
  transition period, 86–87
  vegans, 97
  see also Diet; Health

Obesity, 104, 111–112; *see also* Weight loss
Occupational differences, 32–33
Organic foods, 146–147
Organizations
  lifestyle, 163–165
  listing of, 267–268
  social relations, 186
  transition period, 78–79
Ovo-vegetarians, 33

Pain, 24–26, 77
Parenting, *see* Child rearing
Peace movement, 27–29, 48–49, 118–119
Personal growth motives, 45–46
Pets, 73, 161–163; *see also* Animal rights
Pick, Philip, 17
Plato, 2
Porphyry, 27
Pregnancy, 8
Prisons, 167–168
Processed foods, 141–142
Protein, 6–8
Protein complementarity, 7–8
Psychological change, 116–126
  negative, 123–126
  positive, 117–123

Regan, Tom, 24, 68–69
Religion
  animal rights, 26–27
  health, 5
  history, 3, 4
  motivation, 40–44
  spiritual changes, 126–129
  transition period, 78
  vegetarianism, 15–18
Restaurants, 153–157
Riboflavin, 8, 222

Salmonellosis, 14
Schools, 236
Self-development, 45–46
Serotonin, 121–122
Seventh-Day Adventists, 5, 18, 42
Sex role and sex differences, 33
  child rearing, 230
  dating, 205–206
  intimate relationships, 219–221
  weight loss, 111–112
Sexuality, 129–131; *see also* Intimate relationships; Marriage
Shatner, William, 80
Shelley, Percy Bysshe, 4
Shopping, 144–146
Siblings, 234
Singer, Isaac Bashevis, 28
Singer, Peter, 21, 23, 24, 68

Slaughter, 74–76, 80; *see also* Animal rights
Social conformity, 52
Social forces, 64–68
Social justice, 27–29
Social relations, 182–199
  child rearing, 224, 232–237
  conflict avoidance, 246–250
  defensive nonvegetarians, 194–196
  dining with nonvegetarians, 190–194
  extended visits, 197–199
  friends' reactions, 192–195
  lapsed vegetarians, 252–254
  living arrangements, 196–197
  missionary attitude of vegetarians, 201–204
  problems in, 187–190
  stereotyping, 199–201
  vegetarian friends, 186–187
  see also Intimate relationships
Soy products, 139
Spirituality
  fasting, 148–149
  well-being, 126–129
  see also Religion
Sri Chinmoy, 42
Stereotyping, 199–201
Stress, 122
Surgery, 77

Tempeh, 139
Theory of evolution, 3–4, 25–26
Thoreau, Henry David, 29
Tobacco, 149–150, 258, 261, 263
Tofu, 139
Tolstoy, Leo, 4
Topsoil, 19–20
Trace elements, 8
Transition period, 63–101
  dietary change, 94–98
  difficulties in, 88–94
  effectuation, 81–84
  films, 79–81
  initial influences, 63–81
Transition period (*cont.*)
  media, 68–70
  organizations, 78–79
  personal experience, 70–78
  preparedness, 84–87
  social forces, 64–68
  veganism, 98–101
  see also Motivation
Travel, 157–160

U.S. Department of Health and Human Services, 12

Vegans
  family response to, 176, 180
  transition, 98–101
VEGEDINE, 242
Vegetarian communities, 165–166, 187
Vegetarianism
  animal rights movement, 21–27
  environmentalism and, 18–21
  future of, 259–266
  health considerations, 5–15
  history of, 2–5
  longevity, 14
  motivation, v, 1, 31–61
  popularity of, 1–2
  religion and, 15–18
  sex role and, 219–221
  social justice and peace movements, 27–29
  transition to, 63–101; *see also* Transition period
  variety of foods, 137–138
Vegetarian lifestyle, *see* Lifestyle
Vegetarians
  characteristics of, 32–34
  identification of, 31–32
  lapsed, 252–259
  missionary attitude and tactics, 201–204, 250–252
  sex role, 219–221
  stereotypes, 199–201
  variety among, vi–viii
  views of, 56–61

Vegetarian Society, 4–5
Vitamin B-12, 9–10, 97, 114–115, 222
Vitamin D, 9
Vitamins
  children, 222
  colds, 107
  deficiency of, 114–115
  nutrition, 8–10
  vegans, 97

Water resources, 19, 20
Weight loss
  improvements in, 111–112
  sexuality, 129, 130
  see also Obesity
Well-being, 103–136
  evaluation of former self, 131–135
Well-being (*cont.*)
  future, 264–265
  health, 103–116
  psychological changes, 116–126
  sexual changes, 129–131
  spiritual changes, 126–129
  see also Health
White, Ellen, 18
Wishaw, Ian, 25
World hunger, 47–48
Wurtman, Judith, 107

Yoga, 77–78
Youthfulness, 112–113

Zen Buddhism, 16, 28
Zinc, 8, 222